Primer of Polysomnogram Interpretation

Primer of Polysomnogram Interpretation

MARK R. PRESSMAN, Ph.D., Dipl. A.B.S.M.

*Clinical Professor of Medicine, Jefferson Medical College, Philadelphia;
Director of Sleep Medicine Services, Division of Pulmonary
and Critical Care Medicine, Department of Medicine,
The Lankenau Hospital, Wynnewood, Pennsylvania and
Paoli Memorial Hospital, Paoli, Pennsylvania*

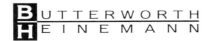

Boston   Oxford   Aukland   Johannesburg   Melbourne   New Delhi

Library of Congress Cataloging-in-Publication Data

Pressman, Mark R.
     Primer of polysomnogram interpretation / Mark R. Pressman.
          p. ; cm.
     Includes bibliographical references and index.
     ISBN 0-7506-9782-2 (HC : alk. paper)
     1. Sleep disorders. 2. Polysomnography. I. Title.
     [DNLM: 1. Sleep Disorders—diagnosis. 2. Polysomnography. 3. Sleep Disorders—therapy. 4. Sleep Stages. WM 188 P935p 2002]
     RC547 .P74 2002
     616.8′498—dc21

                                                                2001037713

British Library Cataloguing-in-Publication Data
A catalogue record for this book is available from the British Library.

The publisher offers special discounts on bulk orders of this book.
For information, please contact:

Manager of Special Sales
Butterworth-Heinemann
225 Wildwood Avenue
Woburn, MA 01801-2041
Tel: 781-904-2500
Fax: 781-904-2620

For information on all Butterworth–Heinemann publications available, contact our World Wide Web home page at: http://www.bh.com

10 9 8 7 6 5 4 3 2 1

Printed in the United States of America

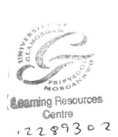

For Art Spielman, Ph.D., mentor and friend,
who had the good sense not to fire me after my first
really shaky night in the sleep laboratory. But for this act
of kindness and restraint, I would probably be
flipping burgers somewhere.

In memory of my cousin Isaac Ledor, ז"ל,
old world gentleman, good guy, and holocaust survivor.

For my mother Sylviette, determined and graceful
under pressure, and my father Walter, still doing
The New York Times *crossword puzzle in pen.*

For my wife Rosalie and children Ariel and Gabriel
who have patiently listened to me say, "It's almost done,"
lo these many years.

Contents

Figures and Tables

Preface

I was very lucky to have started my career in sleep medicine as a staff member of the Sleep/Wake Disorders Center at Montefiore Hospital in the Bronx, New York. In the late 1970s I was both research assistant/technician and graduate student. I completed my doctoral dissertation in the Center's sleep laboratory when it wasn't being used for patients. Sleep medicine was then in its infancy and it seemed that we would learn something new from almost every patient.

The highlight of my time there was the weekly working case conference, which I tried never to miss. Every patient who had had a sleep study and some who didn't had their cases reviewed in detail. Each case conference was attended by as many as ten physicians, psychologists, technicians, and students. Usually, the attending physician for each case, which included such notable sleep experts as Charles Pollak, Elliot Weitzman, Daniel Wagner, Richard Ferber, and Michael Thorpy, presented first, followed by Arthur Spielman, a clinical psychologist who had also seen every patient. The paper polysomnographic record was then placed on the conference table and presented along with the summary statistics. Most often this was done by Peter McGregor, first president of the Association of Polysomnographic Technologists. Often, case conference attendees would page through the polysomnographic record and argue over its contents. A freewheeling discussion then ensued that could last for 30 minutes or more, especially if our department chairman, Elliot Weitzman, was in attendance and was interested in some aspect of the case. Usually the discussion resulted in a final diagnosis and a plan of treatment that had the support of the group.

Looking back, I believe those case conference discussions have shaped my thinking to this day. The case conference was a *process* by which Sleep/Wake Disorders Center staff evaluated evidence and made decisions. Everything was taken into consideration. The polysomnogram played an important role, but was almost always secondary to clinical history, skills, knowledge, and wisdom. The modern day sleep medicine specialist does not always have access to a case conference or even other sleep specialists who could assist in reviewing case materials. Nevertheless, the individual sleep specialist can still follow the same process of collecting, reviewing, and evaluating all case material before arriving at a decision. This book is an attempt to provide a starting point for individuals who wish to learn one aspect of this important process.

M.R.P.

Acknowledgments

This book is the result of several years of case material collection, writing, and terrible writer's block. It could not have happened without the continuous support and patience of many people. I am most grateful to Susan Pioli of Butterworth–Heinemann who first agreed to publish this book as my editor, and has risen to Director of Medical Publishing while waiting for this book to be finished. I appreciate the years of support and her infinite patience. The patience and assistance of my other editorial and production editors, Jennifer Rhuda and Jodie Allen, are much appreciated.

My wife Rosalie has been a source of constant and understanding support. Additionally, I want to thank Art Spielman and his crew of graduate students for early reviews of some of the material that appears in this book.

Introduction

The interpretation of polysomnographic (PSG) data is the end point of a complicated process. It does not and should not start with a review of the summary statistics. All information, including the patient's medical, psychological, and sleep histories; laboratory orientation, calibration, and preparation of equipment; patient hook-up and calibration; acquisition of 8–16 channels of physiological data; review of sleep log; lights out and lights on questionnaires; scoring of physiological data for sleep stages, respiration, movements, ECG, and other data, need to be reviewed by the interpreter. All prior technical and professional elements of the patient evaluation can have a bearing on the interpretation of the sleep study.

The job of interpreting the polysomnogram requires a wide variety of skills and knowledge. The PSG interpreter must be familiar with how to record and analyze EEGs, EOGs, EMGs of several types, ECGs, respiration of several types as well as other physiological variables. Further, the interrelationship of these variables must be understood from moment to moment, across the night and in the summary data. The PSG interpreter is thus a jack of many interpreting skills.

In interpreting the PSG, it is important to evaluate not only whether data deviates from published statistical norms but also whether it is clinically significant. Summary data can deviate from established norms quite significantly but not be clinically significant or account for the patient's presenting complaint. On the other hand, data may appear within normal limits but still be clinically significant. The interpreter's clinical judgment and knowledge of the patient's complaint is at least as important to proper interpretation and diagnosis as the published norms.

This book focuses on the *process* of interpreting polysomnographic data, with emphasis on sleep parame-

ters. I like to think that this primer, in some small way, will put the *sleep* back into sleep studies. This volume is not intended to be an all-encompassing handbook or encyclopedia with answers for every situation. That would clearly be an impossible task. In 1997 alone, over 2,000 articles with sleep or sleep disorders as the main topic appeared in professional medical, psychological, or scientific journals in addition to numerous books. Many of these articles and books are potential sources of information, useful in the interpretation of polysomnograms and the diagnosis of sleep disorders. Rather, this volume is a primer, providing basic techniques, information, and guidance about possible ways of looking at and understanding data that can be used by the sleep disorders clinician in pursuit of the correct interpretation and diagnosis. No single book or black box computer system is capable of providing all of the answers. Rather, only the well-trained and educated sleep specialist ultimately can come to the right decisions.

GENERAL CONSIDERATIONS

1. All PSG data summary terms discussed are common summary parameters thought to reflect some important aspect of the patient's sleep. Many sleep disorders clinicians have developed specialized ways of summarizing data in addition to the more common terminology. These summary terms cannot be reviewed in this volume.

2. All comments regarding interpretation of sleep related parameters assume that sleep was visually analyzed according to the rules of the Rechtschaffen and Kales manual.[1] Despite occasional controversies, this manual remains the standard method

for analyzing sleep. In an editorial in *Sleep*, Roehr and Carskadon wrote:

> The Rechtschaffen and Kales manual provided the field with criteria which has made possible the achievement of high reliability in sleep-stage scoring both within and between laboratories. It also established a standard terminology which has been used by sleep scientists to communicate their findings over the ensuing years. In specifying *standard* techniques for use in recording human sleep, the manual also provided a basis by which sleep scientists could communicate *deviations* in technique, which in turn has led to relevant discoveries regarding changes in sleep over the age span (e.g., delta amplitude in childhood vs aging). Standard descriptions of normal sleep then began to serve as a backdrop for the recognition of various sleep pathologies, and this in turn illuminated the need for standardized scoring criteria for transient changes in sleep state that the Rechtschaffen and Kales manual was not designed to address.[2(p. 445)]

Further, the American Academy of Sleep Medicine mandates its use in all accredited sleep disorders centers. For these reasons, the PSG interpreter should be expert at its use. For the remainder of this volume, the Rechtschaffen and Kales manual will be referred to with its universally used abbreviation R&K.

3. All suggestions and comments regarding the interpretation of sleep, respiratory, movement-related, and other data are based on published papers and chapters as well as my 20 years of experience in making sense of all the squiggly lines. Therefore, some comments will reflect my personal biases.

4. Interpretation of PSGs can be done only in the proper context. That context requires knowledge of the patient's general medical, psychological, and sleep history. Additionally, the patient's subjective report about the quality and quantity of sleep in the sleep laboratory during polysomnographic testing is essential.

5. Interpreters who do not actually perform the sleep staging, respiratory analysis, and other types of analyses used to create the summary PSG report,

at a minimum, must review the raw data and verify the accuracy and completeness of the scoring.

6. Interpreters who rely on others to do the initial scoring of the PSG should be familiar with scorers' preferences and prejudices and establish summary data parameters for the scorer.

7. Summary data sheets may not always provide a good reflection of what actually occurred in the sleep recording. The majority of epoch (MOE) scoring rule that is an essential part of R&K scoring necessitates a drastic reduction in data across the night, so that large quantities of data can be handled easily. However, sometimes the baby is indeed thrown out with the bathwater as part of the scoring process. It is the interpreter's duty to make sure the PSG summary and interpretation are an accurate and valid reflection of what occurred during the sleep recording. Only in this way can a proper interpretation and diagnosis be made.

GENERAL ALGORITHM FOR PSG INTERPRETATION

- Review patient history for symptoms and presenting complaints. What symptoms or complaints are you trying to confirm, account for, or rule out with the PSG?
- Review raw data in the sleep recording.
- Review the sleep technologist's notes.
- Review the patient PM and AM questionnaires.
- Determine the age- and sex-related range of values thought to be normal, if available.
- Review sleep log: Determine the patient's usual time in bed and the estimated total sleep time, number of awakenings, and the usual bedtime and wake time.
- Compare the values in the PSG to normative data and the patient's estimates.
- Explain any discrepancies.
- Determine what values in the PSG summary are artifacts of the sleep laboratory and what values are representative of the patient's usual sleep.
- Review the recording for other features that may have clinical significance.
- Review the videotape for sleep-related behaviors, if necessary.
- Make a final statement as to likely interpretation and diagnosis.

1

Interpretation of Polysomnographic Data

NORMAL SLEEP PARAMETERS

Sleep data have been collected on various groups of research subjects and patients for more than 30 years. However, a set of generally accepted norms for sleep quantity and quality does not exist. All reported "normative data" appear to suffer from some methodological problem, be it sample size, recording technique, medication, failure to screen for sleep disorders, or the like. However, by looking at a variety of studies reporting purportedly normal data, it is possible to get a good general idea of the normal range of sleep quantity and quality. Tables 1-1 through 1-8 present selected samples of normal sleep data from the sleep literature. Additional data are presented on the type of sample, method of data collection, and so forth to aid the interpreter in assessing the validity, reliability, and clinical usefulness of this data in the interpretation of polysomnograms (PSGs).

The concept of "normative data" is statistical and may not have clinical significance. A patient's total sleep time may be three standard deviations below or above the mean values presented in the normative data, a statistically rare finding, but have no effect on his or her daytime alertness, cognitive functioning, mental status, or activities of daily living. Therefore, normative data must be used judiciously, with the possibility that deviations from it may not produce meaningful clinical consequences.

The interpreter of sleep data must decide if the point of comparison is to be the patient's first night in the sleep laboratory versus the first or second night recorded in the sleep research laboratory as normative data. The second night recorded in the sleep research laboratory may represent values closer to the every night values expected of patients in certain categories. However, first night data as recorded in the sleep research laboratory may represent a more realistic point of comparison, as most clinical patients spend only one night in the sleep laboratory. Because of the possibility of first night effect (FNE), many clinical patients may not sleep as well in the sleep laboratory as at home. However, this may depend on the subject's level of comfort while in the sleep laboratory.

THE MAJORITY OF EPOCH RULE AND POLYSOMNOGRAM INTERPRETATION

All sleep data, normal or otherwise, is influenced by the way it is collected and analyzed. One of the most important influences on sleep data is the majority of epoch (MOE) rule. As delineated in Rechtshaffen and Kales,[1] all sleep data are analyzed in epochs of 20 or 30 seconds. Using R&K principles, each epoch receives a single sleep stage score. However, sleep stages, especially when recorded in the clinical sleep laboratory, often do not occur in long homogeneous stretches. A single epoch may contain two or three sleep stages, but only one sleep stage may be scored, based on the majority of the epoch rule. In cases in which there are repetitive arousals from sleep, such as in sleep apnea, the majority of the epoch rule may result in a considerable underscoring or overscoring of wakefulness or stage 1 sleep, depending on which is the majority and which is in the minority. When transient stage 1 sleep is underscored because it occupies the minority of the 30-second epoch, total sleep time is likely to be low. A low total sleep time (TST) not only gives a false impression of low sleep quantity and sleep efficiency, but as TST is

TABLE 1-1
Normal Sleep in Men Ages 20–29, 30–39, 40–49, 50–59, and over 60 Years

	Age (Years)									
	20–29 (N = 44)		30–39 (N = 23)		40–49 (N = 49)		50–59 (N = 41)		>60 (N = 29)	
	Mean	*SD*	*Mean*	*SD*	*Mean*	*SD*	*Mean*	*SD*	*Mean*	*SD*
Total time in bed	404.9	44.1	393.1	58.2	404.2	49.4	393.0	51.1	395.7	42.8
Total sleep time	347.3	62.5	340.0	70.8	329.4	54.6	331.6	63.6	298.4	61.3
Total wake time	57.6	61.0	53.1	48.3	74.9	46.7	61.4	44.7	97.3	50.5
Stage 1 (min)	16.4	11.5	13.1	8.2	21.9	13.0	22.0	13.0	24.4	14.1
Stage 1 (%)	4.1	3.0	3.4	2.1	5.4	3.3	5.5	3.0	6.1	3.5
Stage 2 (min)	197.0	42.4	195.8	48.2	208.8	50.2	212.6	48.6	202.5	44.7
Stage 2 (%)	48.7	9.2	49.7	10.0	51.8	11.7	54.2	10.2	51.0	9.1
Stage 3 + 4 (SWS) (min)	61.9	22.1	58.4	28.5	34.6	31.3	27.9	26.3	19.3	16.4
Stage 3 + 4 (SWS) (%)	15.5	7.3	15.2	8.4	8.6	8.9	7.1	8.0	5.1	5.7
REM (min)	72.0	29.2	72.7	35.9	64.2	27.5	69.0	24.7	52.2	23.9
REM (%)	17.8	7.1	18.2	7.9	15.8	6.4	17.6	5.9	13.2	5.7
Sleep efficiency (%)	86.2	14.2	86.4	11.6	81.7	10.8	84.3	11.1	75.4	13.2
Sleep latency	11.8	13.1	13.4	10.1	14.2	14.0	8.7	11.4	15.3	14.9
Total no. of awakenings	9.6	8.2	7.7	4.2	11.6	5.3	11.4	4.5	14.1	6.7
Awakening index (per hr sleep)	1.5	1.2	1.3	0.8	1.8	0.8	1.8	0.7	2.2	1.0
Stage shifts	47.1	23.6	39.9	11.8	46.7	18.8	46.3	12.7	50.8	21.9

Sample size: 23–49 per group, 218 total subjects (Tables 1-2 and 1-4 combined).

Age range: 20–60+ years.

Sex: Men only.

Scoring technique: R&K.

Number of consecutive nights of recording: 2.

Source: Modified from Hirshkowitz M, Moore CA, Hamilton CR, Rando KC, Karacan I. Polysomnography of adults and elderly: Sleep architecture, respiration, and leg movement. *Journal of Clinical Neurophysiology.* 1992;9(1):56–62.

used to compute indexes such as the respiratory disturbance index (RDI), an abnormally low TST may result in a drastically and even ridiculously elevated RDI. When this occurs an explanation or caution should be added to the interpretation. For example,

Although large numbers of obstructive sleep apneas are present in this recording, the respiratory disturbance index of 243/hr of sleep is a methodological artifact. The standard conventions of sleep staging require each 30-second epoch of sleep to be characterized by the sleep stage that occupies the majority of that epoch. In this recording, the patient was awakened repetitively by short apneas and hypopneas after less than 15 seconds of sleep elapsed. Therefore, wakefulness most often formed the majority of scoring epochs, severely reducing total sleep time

used to compute the respiratory disturbance index. When the RDI was computed using total recording time, the RDI was 62/hr, still consistent with severe obstructive sleep apnea.

The tables of normative data are presented as potential points of comparison for PSG interpreter.

NORMAL SLEEP QUOTA, OR HOW MUCH IS ENOUGH?

How much sleep does an individual need? This unexpectedly controversial topic has been argued over since well before the appearance of modern sleep medicine or sleep research. Sleep experts and grandmothers have offered their opinions, sometimes without much more evidence.

TABLE 1-2

Normal Sleep in Men and Women Ages 30–39 and 61–81 Years

	30–39 Years		61–81 Years	
	Mean	*SD*	*Mean*	*SD*
Total recording time (min)	404.0	46	422.0	58
Total sleep time (min)	386.0	40	364.0	47
Sleep efficiency (%)	95.5	3.1	86.4	7.4
Wake time (%)	4.4	3.2	13.7	7.3
Stage 1 (%)	5.7	2.7	11.3	4.8
Stage 2 (%)	45.5	3.3	42.6	6.8
Stage 3 + 4 (SWS) (%)	27.1	3.4	18.7	8.7
REM sleep (%)	21.1	3.5	14.9	4.6
Wake after sleep onset	10.7	11.0	46.1	34.8

Study purpose: Compare sleep of older and younger subjects.

Sample size: Total 23, 11 in older group, 12 in younger group.

Age range: Group 1, mean age 68.4 ± 4.0 men, 69.5 ± 2.1 women; group 2, mean age, men 33.2 ± 1.5, women 34.7 ± 1.2 years.

Sex: Group 1 = 5 women, 6 men; group 2 = 6 men, 6 women

Subject selection criteria: General good health, reported selves to be "good sleepers," nonsmokers, no history of alcohol abuse.

Subject exclusion criteria: Older group was free of cardiorespiratory disorders and other major disorders following physician's exam.

Medication: Not noted.

Scoring technique: R&K.

Number of nights of recording: 4.

Number of night reported: 2.

Source: Modified from Naifeh KH, Severinghaus JW, Kamiya J. Effects of aging on sleep-related changes in respiratory variables. *Sleep.* 1987;10(2):160–171.

TABLE 1-3

Normal Sleep Quantity and Quality in the Elderly

	Mean	*SD*	*Range*
Total recording time (min)	552.0	39	463–558
Total sleep time (min)	426.0	75	250–534
Wake after sleep onset	126.0	68	25–265
Sleep efficiency (%)	72.0	12	43–93
Stage 1 (min)	100.0	35	34–169
Stage 1 (%)	18.0	5.8	9.1–30.1
Stage 2 (min)	218.0	50	121–309
Stage 2 (%)	39.0	8.9	23.7–55.0
Stage 3 (min)	22.0	16	0–47
Stage 3 (%)	5.3	6.7	0–10.2
Stage 4 (min)	15.0	19	0–57
Stage 4 (%)	2.7	3.5	0–14
REM (min)	72.0	32	11–147
REM (%)	13.1	5.8	1.9–25.1
Sleep latency (min)	19.0	19	2–98
Transient arousals	160	104	24–373
Transient arousal index	23	15	3–54

Study purpose: Examine the relationship between sleep fragmentation and daytime alertness in a group of elderly subjects.

Subjects: 12 women, mean age 73.4 (range 65–82 years), and 12 men, mean age 72.3 years (range 63–86).

Subject selection criteria: No complaints of sleep disorders or daytime sleepiness.

Subject exclusion criteria: Must be fully ambulatory and in good health.

Medication: Not noted.

Scoring technique: R&K.

Nights recorded: 2.

Source: Modified from Carskadon MA, Brown ED, Dement WC. Sleep fragmentation in the elderly: Relationship to daytime sleep tendency. *Neurobiology of Aging.* 1982;3:321–327.

It is clear that the question of how much sleep a patient *needs* is not the same question as how much sleep is statistically normal for a patient of a certain age, sex, and so on.

The question of how much sleep a patient needs often turns on how much sleep is necessary for the patient to awaken refreshed, feel alert during the day, and perform at a reasonably high level. Theoretically and practically, one patient may function well with only 6 hours of sleep, while another might appear severely sleepy. This makes the practical and clinical significance of normal sleep studies and their application to the task of interpreting diagnostic PSGs uncertain.

TABLE 1-4

Comparison of Normal Sleep in Healthy Young (21–30 years) and Elderly (81–90 years) Subjects

| | 21–30 Years | | 81–90 Years | |
	Mean	SD	Mean	SD
Total sleep time (min)	426.0	39	368.0	50
Sleep efficiency (%)	93.3	4.0	76.8	10.8
Wake after sleep onset (min)	10	14	85	49
Sleep latency (min)	19	13	28	31
Stage 3 + 4 (SWS) (%)	16.0	7.3	3.7	5.2
REM (%)	26.1	4.2	20.1	5.4
REM sleep latency	66	39	58	50

Age spans the "21–30 Years" and "81–90 Years" column groups.

Subjects: Group 1 consisted of 16 men and 18 women with a mean age of 83.1 years (range 81–90), group 2 consisted of 9 men and 21 women with a mean age of 25.5 years (range 21–30).

Subject selection criteria: Generally healthy.

Subject exclusion criteria: No history of sleep disorders.

Subject inclusion criteria: Healthy with no psychiatric symptoms. Vigorous and community dwelling.

Medication: No medication known to affect sleep or circadian rhythms.

Recording techniques: R&K.

Scoring technique: R&K with 1 min scoring epochs, REM sleep latency from onset of stage 2 sleep.

Number of nights of recording: 2.

Night of recording reported: 2.

Source: Modified from Monk TH, Reynolds CF, Buysse DJ, Hoch CC, Jarrett DB, Jennings JR, Kupfer DJ. Circadian characteristics of healthy 80-yr-olds and their relationship to objectively recorded sleep. *Journal of Gerontology: Medical Sciences*. 1991;46(3):171–175.

TABLE 1-5

Normal Sleep in Young (20–29 years) and Elderly (70–79 years) Groups

| | 20–29 Years | | 70–79 Years | |
	Mean	SD	Mean	SD
Total recording time (min)	445	24	507	56
Total sleep time (min)	432	22	470	47
No. of awakenings	1.1	0.8	8.4	5.5
Sleep efficiency (%)	96.0	2.0	82.0	9.0
Stage 1 (% TST)	4.0	2.0	7.0	2.0
Stage 2 (% TST)	52.0	6.0	52.0	8.0
Stage 3 (% TST)	5.0	2.0	6.0	4.0
Stage 4 (% TST)	12.0	6.0	4.0	6.0
REM (% TST)	25.0	4.0	19.0	4.0

Age spans the "20–29 Years" and "70–79 Years" column groups.

Subjects: Two groups of women: the first consisting of subjects 20–29 years; the second, subjects aged 70–79 years. Number of subjects not reported.

Source: Modified from Quan SF, Bamford CR, Beutler LE. Sleep disturbances in the elderly. *Geriatrics*. 1984;39(9):42–47.

TABLE 1-6

Normal Sleep in Healthy Middle-Aged and Elderly Subjects (58–82 years)

	58–82 Years	
	Mean	Standard Deviation
Total recording time (min)	438.8	35.6
Total sleep time (min)	368.7	44.5
Total wake time (min)	47.4	32.8
Sleep efficiency (%)	84.1	8.3
Stage 1 (%)	9.7	8.2
Stage 2 (%)	64.9	8.3
Stage 3+4 (%)	2.5	3.9
REM (%)	20.2	24.9
Sleep latency (min)	22.2	16.9
REM latency (min)	57.6	16.9
No. of arousals	6.8	2.7

Study Purpose: Compare sleep of elderly depressed, demented, and healthy.

Subjects: Healthy subjects include 8 men and 17 women with a mean age of 69.0 ± 5.0 (range 58–82).

Subject selection criteria: Healthy subjects had no history of psychiatric illness and no sleep complaints. No history of active disease and normal laboratory values.

Recording techniques: Standard.

Recording location: Sleep research laboratory.

Scoring technique: Modified R&K, 1 min epochs, use of intermediate stage 2 with poor sleep spindles and k-complexes. Sleep latency to first sleep spindle.

No. of consecutive nights of recording: 3.

Data reported from nights: Mean of 2 + 3.

Source: Modified from Reynolds CF, Kupfer DJ, Taska LS, Hoch CC, Spiker DG, Sewitch DE, Zimmer B, Marin RS, Nelson JP, Martin D, Morycyz R. EEG sleep in elderly depressed, demented and healthy subjects. *Biological Psychiatry.* 1985;20:431–442.

TABLE 1-7

Sleep in Middle-Aged and Older Patients with Sleep Complaints

	Age			
	Mean Age, 66 Years		Mean Age, 42 Years	
	Minutes	Standard Deviation	Minutes	Standard Deviation
Total sleep time (min)	324.0	13.0	408.0	5.2
Total wake time (min)	155.0	11.0	102.0	4.0
Sleep latency (min)	24.0	3.7	23.0	2.4
Number of awakenings >2 min	9.3	0.7	8.6	1.6
Stage 3 (min)	23.0	2.9	29.0	1.2
Stage 4 (min)	24.0	3.8	36.0	2.6
REM (min)	49.0	3.3	72.0	1.8

Study purpose: Compare the quality and quantity of sleep in younger and older patients undergoing evaluation for a sleep disorder in a sleep disorders center.

Subjects: 83 patients with a mean age of 66 ± 0.6 years and 423 patients with a mean age of 42 ± 0.6 years. Patients had a very mixed group of final sleep disorder diagnoses including disorders of excessive daytime sleepiness and insomnia.

Subject selection criteria: All patients during 1978–1979 who completed their evaluations at the Stanford Sleep Disorders Clinic. All patients discontinued hypnotic medications 2 weeks prior to study.

Subject exclusion criteria: None.

Scoring technique: R&K.

Source: Modified from Coleman RM, Miles LE, Guilleminualt CC, Zarcone VP, van den Hoed J, Dement WC. Sleep-wake disorders in the elderly: A polysomnographic analysis. *Journal of the American Geriatrics Society.* 1981;29(7):289–296.

TABLE 1-8
Sleep Parameters in a Large Group of Randomly Selected
Subjects (30–60 years)

	Women (N = 250)		Men (N = 352)	
	Mean	Standard Deviation	Mean	Standard Deviation
Total sleep time (min)	358.7	71.0	333.7	58.9
Stage 1 (%)	8.2	4.6	11.0	6.3
Stage 2 (%)	60.0	10.0	63.0	10.0
Stage 3 + 4 (%)	13.0	8.5	8.9	7.6
REM (%)	18.0	6.2	17.0	6.0

Study purpose: Determine the incidence of sleep-disordered breathing in a randomly selected group of middle-aged adults.

Subjects: 602 employed men and women, aged 30–60 years.

Subject exclusion criteria: Unstable cardiopulmonary disease, upper airway disease, or recent surgery.

Medication: Not noted.

Scoring technique: R&K.

Source: Modified from Young T, Palta M, Dempsey J, Skatrud J, Weber S, Badr S. The occurrence of sleep disordered breathing among the middle-aged. *New England Journal of Medicine.* 1993; 328:1230–1235.

2

General Factors

POTENTIAL EFFECTS OF PRIOR LIMITATIONS OF SLEEP QUANTITY OR QUALITY

Partial Acute or Partial Cumulative Sleep Deprivation

The accurate interpretation of a night of polysomnography requires data on the patient's sleep quantity, quality, and timing for at least one week prior to the scheduled sleep study to determine if the sleep recording is typical of the patient's usual sleep. Partial sleep deprivation can have significant effects both on nocturnal sleep variables and daytime sleepiness (see Figure 6-1). A voluntarily restricted sleep schedule can have the following effects:

- Preservation of rapid eye movement (REM) and deep sleep minutes with increased percentage of REM sleep and stage 3 and 4 sleep, due to decreased overall total sleep time.[3]
- Decreased wakefulness and stage 1 sleep.
- Rebound sleep (Table 2-1) may result if the patient abandons a restricted sleep schedule due to sleep laboratory request or absence of usual cues (e.g., work, family) that are important in maintaining the restricted schedule.

TABLE 2-1
Rebound Sleep Values Following Total Sleep Deprivation for 40 or 64 Hours

	Young Adults (40 hr; % change from baseline)	Older Adults (40 hr; % change from baseline)	Older Normals (64 hr; % change from baseline)	Older Insomniacs (64 hr; % change from baseline)
Sleep latency	38, +9			
Wake %	44, +19	51, +11		
Stage 1 %	42, +10	59, +14	56	52
Stage 2 %	87, +10	95, +7	107	120
Slow-wave sleep	153, +11	156, +23	236	330
REM	89, +13	104, +9	26	92
REM latency	101, +20	77, +20	35	96

Note: Rebound sleep on first recovery night after one night (40 hr wakefulness) or two nights (64 hr wakefulness) of complete sleep deprivation. The percent increase or decrease from baseline indicates change compared to baseline nights. Percentages <100% indicate a reduction in variable compared to baseline and percentages >100% indicate an increase compared to baseline. Standard deviation included when more than one study was available.

Source: Modified from Bonnet MH. Sleep deprivation. In Kryger MH, Roth T, Dement WC (eds). *Principles and Practice of Sleep Medicine.* Philadelphia: Saunders, 1994:62.

Sleep Fragmentation or Poor Sleep Quality

Sleep deprivation comes in a variety of forms. One of the least understood and potentially most important forms of sleep deprivation is sleep fragmentation, especially when sleep is fragmented by relatively brief interruptions. Recent research has shown that interruptions in sleep, often called *arousals*, may be too short for the patient to be conscious of or remember in the morning but nevertheless have a significant impact on the refreshing quality of sleep, performance, and daytime alertness later that day. Sleep quality is every bit as important as sleep quantity. It is possible to sleep for eight or more hours in a night and still awaken feeling sleepy, groggy, or unrefreshed, if sleep quality is poor. A variety of published experimental and clinical research has found that sleep fragmentation produces measurable changes in daytime alertness, cognitive functioning, psychosocial functioning (Table 2-2). At higher levels, sleep fragmentation may produce performance deficits similar to those found after long periods of total sleep deprivation (see also Table 4-1 for the effects of sleep fragmentation caused by sleep-disordered breathing). Decrements in daytime alertness and performance can occur at relatively mild levels of sleep fragmentation.

TABLE 2-2

Effects of Experimental Sleep Fragmentation

Arousals per Hour	Source of Arousals	Type of Arousals	Description	Reference
6	Tone	Ss required to respond	After two nights of sleep fragmentation, significant decrements in performance measures, but not as severe as in 60/hr rate. "Periods of uninterrupted sleep in excess of 10 minutes are required for sleep to be restorative" (p. 263) (young adults 18–28 yr)	4
8.5	Tone	EEG-based arousal	After two nights of fragmentation, MSLT decreased from mean of 12.9 ± 4.8 to 8.5 ± 2.0 (young adults, mean 25.8 yr)	5
14	Tone	Ss required to respond	After two nights of sleep fragmentation (10 min continuous sleep followed by 20 min disrupted sleep), significant decrements in performance measures	6
14	Various tones	EEG arousal	After two nights of sleep fragmentation, significantly reduced sleep latencies on MSLT (14.3 ± 3.6 vs. 9.5 ± 5 min)	7
30	Tone	Ss required to respond	After two nights of sleep fragmentation, vigilance performance and nap latency (single AM nap) decreased compared to baseline; no different from group required to have EEG arousal only	8
30	Tone	EEG arousal	After two nights of sleep fragmentation, vigilance performance and nap latency (single AM nap) decreased compared to baseline; no different from group required to respond behaviorally	8
30	Tones	EEG arousal for >3 sec	A single night of fragmentation (mean age 24 ± 3 yrs) resulted in statistically significant decreases compared to uninterrupted baseline in MSLT (11 ± 7 vs. 7 ± 2 min) as well as measures of mood, sustained attention, and mental flexibility	9
60	Tone	Ss required to respond	After two nights of sleep fragmentation, significant changes in subjective, behavioral, and EEG measures similar to that found after 40–60 hr total sleep deprivation (young adults 18–32 yr)	9
60	Tone	Ss required to respond	After two nights of sleep fragmentation, significant changes in performance measures equivalent to that found after 40–60 hr total sleep deprivation (young adults 18–28 yr)	4
60	Tones	Change in arterial blood pressure or heart rate with no visible EEG arousal	After single night of sleep fragmentation (mean age 25 ± 6) resulted in a statistically significant decrease compared to uninterrupted baseline in MSLT (8.0 ± 3.1 vs. 6.2 ± 2.1 min) and mood	11

Note: From selected studies that produced fragmented sleep artificially using acoustic stimuli. Studies differ methodologically in significant ways especially in the type and duration of the arousal produced.

Abbreviations: Ss = subjects; MSLT = Multiple Sleep Latency Test.

Sleep Lab Effects: The First Night Effect

First night effect (FNE) is a phenomenon that has its roots in early sleep research. Early on, it was noted that research subjects spending more than one night in the sleep laboratory usually slept worse on the first night than on the second or succeeding nights. The poorer sleep of the first night usually consisted of lower sleep efficiency, more stage 1 sleep, more awakenings, and lower quantities of deep sleep.[11,12] These changes were consistent with the generally held notion that sleeping in a novel environment (e.g., sleep laboratory, hotel room) is likely to result in poorer sleep than usual. Because of the recognition that FNE might prevent recording of normal sleep, research protocols typically require several consecutive nights of recording, often discarding the first night's sleep data and labeling the first night an *adaptation* night.

With the establishment of sleep laboratories to perform diagnostic sleep studies, the concept of FNE was generally accepted as important to an understanding of why patients might not sleep as well in the laboratory as they report sleeping at home. In the early days

of clinical sleep laboratory operation, two nights of sleep recording often were done, with the first night considered to be an "adaptation" night. However, in the modern health care environment, most sleep disorders center laboratories are rarely allowed more than one night to make a diagnosis. Hence, all clinical sleep studies are potentially confounded by FNE.

Early researchers noted in passing that the extent of FNE might be reduced or eliminated if the technical staff was especially courteous or the testing atmosphere comfortable. Compared to the relatively primitive testing facilities used by early sleep researchers, the modern sleep disorders center laboratory sleep room is quite luxurious. The accrediting body for sleep disorders centers, the American Academy of Sleep Medicine (formerly the American Sleep Disorders Association), requires that sleep rooms be relatively large (at least 10 × 14') and furnished like a hotel room. Under these relatively pleasant circumstances, FNE may be minimized. A recent study of patients' reactions to sleep laboratory studies found that most patients described their sleep as typical of sleep at home (Figures 2-1 and 2-2). However, substantial minorities

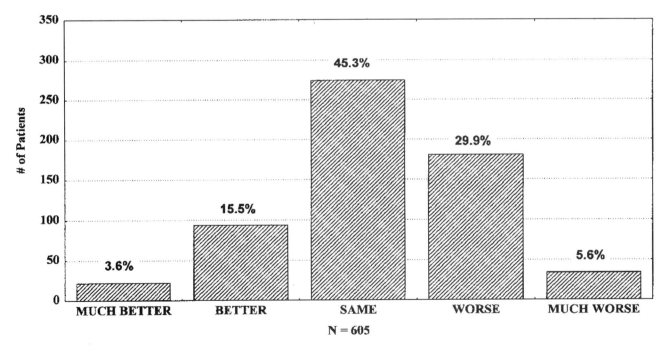

FIGURE 2-1

First night effect and overall comparison to sleep at home. Summary data from a retrospective study of the AM questionnaires of 605 consecutive patients admitted to the sleep disorders center clinical laboratory for diagnostic polysomnograms. All patients were included without regard to medical diagnosis or medication. Results indicate that 35.5% stated that their sleep in the sleep laboratory was worse or much worse than their sleep at home. On the other hand, 19.1% of all patients stated they had slept better or much better than usual in the sleep laboratory. (Reprinted with permission from Pressman MR, Cecere J, Smith B, Peterson DD. Unexpected absence of "first night effect" in many patients undergoing clinical polysomnography: Comparison of patient estimation of laboratory and usual home sleep and alertness. *Sleep Res.* 1995;25:322.)

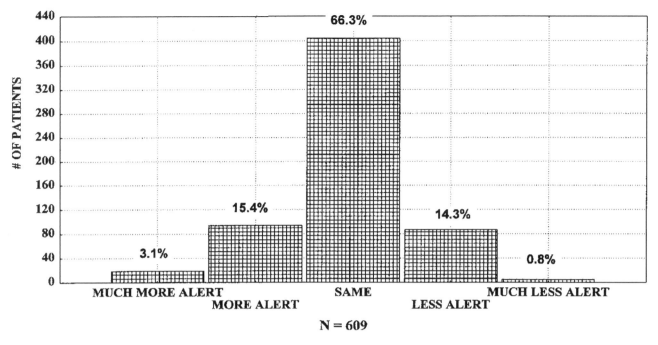

FIGURE 2-2
First night effect and AM alertness. Summary data from a retrospective study of the AM questionnaires of 605 consecutive patients admitted to the sleep disorders center clinical laboratory for diagnostic polysomnograms. All patients were included without regard to medical diagnosis or medication. When asked the more specific question of how alert they felt after awakening from their diagnostic polysomnogram compared to how they usual feel on awakening at home, 15.1% stated they felt less or much less alert while 18.7% reported feeling more alert or much more alert than usual. (Reprinted with permission from Pressman MR, Cecere J, Smith B, Peterson DD. Unexpected absence of "first night effect" in many patients undergoing clinical polysomnography: Comparison of patient estimation of laboratory and usual home sleep and alertness. *Sleep Res.* 1995;25:322.)

of patients described their sleep as either better or worse than sleep at home. The presence of an FNE should not be assumed when reviewing and interpreting clinical sleep data. The interpreter always should consult the patient's morning questionnaire before proceeding to review the summary data.

Of course, many patients still report sleeping worse in the sleep laboratory than at home, and this is easy to understand. Patients who report sleeping better in the sleep laboratory than at home may be harder to understand. This phenomenon, often called *paradoxical* or *reverse first night effect* (PFNE) in the sleep research literature, most often is attributed to patients with a diagnosis of psychophysiological insomnia.[13] These patients find it difficult to sleep in their usual locations (i.e., their own bedrooms) due to negative conditioning and often sleep surprisingly well initially away from their bedrooms, even in the sleep laboratory, electrodes and all. The general conception is that the negative conditioning that makes their own bedrooms such an unpleasant place to sleep does not immediately

generalize to the sleep laboratory. Therefore, the patient may get one or more good nights of sleep away from home. However, if the patient continues to sleep in the new location, the negative conditioning eventually is transferred to the new location and the insomnia returns.

It is clear that many patients without psychophysiological insomnia also sleep better in the sleep laboratory than at home. Often they comment on their morning questionnaires as to how they preferred the bed, mattress, pillow, or blankets of the sleep laboratory. Many patients comment on how much quieter, darker, or safer the sleep laboratory is than their bedroom at home. This may suggest an environmental sleep disorder.

The interpreter of sleep studies must consider the effects of the sleep laboratory on the hoped for typical night of sleep. A review of the PM and AM sleep questionnaires, technologist notes, and even the videotape recording of the patient during sleep may be required. Additionally, the interpreter should consider using normative data collected from the first night of research studies (see Table 1-2).

When Sleep Is Better Than Expected: Rebound Sleep

Many patients studied in the sleep disorders center laboratory are sleep deprived. The sleep deprivation may result from poor prior quantity or quality of sleep. However, when sleep deprivation ends or the sleep fragmenting process is reduced or eliminated—be it from return to a better sleep/wake schedule or elimination of sleep-disordered breathing with nasal continuous positive airway pressure (NCPAP)—both the quantity and quality of sleep may increase well above what is considered normal. Therefore, a research subject who has been totally sleep deprived may show levels of deep sleep and REM sleep 25–100% higher than expected on a "normal" night of sleep. In experimental subjects, deep sleep typically rebounds first followed within a day or two by REM sleep, although this may depend to some degree on whether the time in bed is restricted. REM sleep rebound may follow discontinuation of REM sleep suppressing medications, such as tricyclic antidepressants, MAO inhibitors, amphetamines, or substances of abuse such as alcohol (Table 2-3). REM sleep rebound may continue for weeks after medications are discontinued (Figure 2-3).

Rebound sleep noted in the clinical sleep laboratory almost always has some clinical significance. A higher than expected quantity of deep sleep may indicate that the patient has been recently sleep deprived, perhaps not sleeping well for days or weeks prior to testing. It may indicate that conditions in the sleep laboratory are somehow superior to those at home, permitting sleep to rebound. The elimination of inappropriate noise, light, or disruptive bed partner may permit good quality sleep to return. An unexpectedly high and unexplained percentage of REM sleep may indicate that the patient recently discontinued an undocumented medication or ceased intake of high quantities of alcohol. The patient may have recently changed his or her sleep/wake schedule or moved to a new shift.

A further impact of rebound sleep occurring during a clinical sleep study is that it may confound or camouflage typical sleep patterns or other findings. For example, higher than expected quantities of REM sleep may result in an increase in sleep-disordered breathing, especially for those patients in whom sleep apnea is primarily REM-sleep related. Higher than expected quantities of deep sleep, on the other hand, may have the opposite effect, effectively reducing sleep-disordered breathing.[14] Thus, the presence of rebound sleep during a clinical sleep study may significantly alter the level of severity of the findings and influence treatment options. It also may signify other changes relevant to the final diagnosis.

Rebound sleep may occur when sleep stages are only partially reduced by experimental awakenings or medication effects as well. As with total and partial cumulative sleep deprivation, the sleep debt cannot be discharged until the quantity of the deprived-sleep stage increases above the expected normal amount. This can be seen clearly in Figures 2-4 and 2-5.

Effects of Medication or Withdrawal from Medication

Prescription and over-the-counter (OTC) medications, as well as alcohol, caffeine, and nicotine, can dramatically effect sleep states. These generally can be divided into medications that suppress REM sleep, suppress deep sleep, or result in increased fragmentation of sleep. Withdrawal from these medications can result in significant rebound sleep (see Table 2-2). Withdrawal effects may continue for far longer than expected (see Figure 2-3).

TABLE 2-3
Medication Effects on Sleep

Decrease Sleep Quality	*Decrease Deep Sleep*	*Decrease REM Sleep*
Caffeine	Benzodiazepines*	MAO inhibitors
Nicotine	Central nervous system depressants?	Tricyclic antidepressants
Theophylline		Amphetamines
Amphetamines		Barbiturates
		Alcohol
		Anticholinergics

*Also increase sleep spindle activity (see Table 1-2 and Figure 3-5).

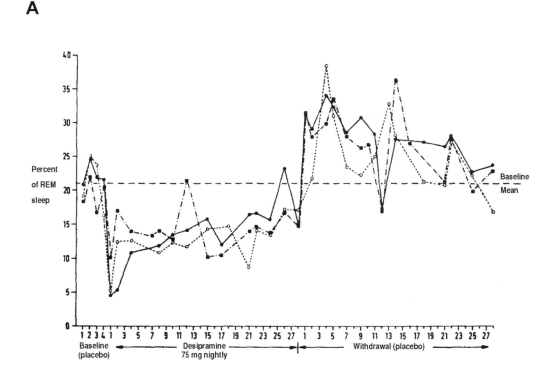

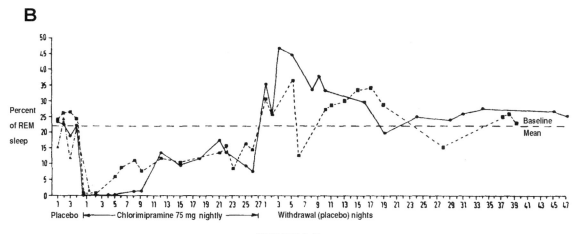

FIGURE 2-3

Treatment and withdrawal from tricyclic antidepressant medications, effects on REM sleep. **(A)** Effects of 75 mg desipramine on three young men. Initial administration resulted in a decrease in REM sleep from 20% at baseline to 5%. Over the next three weeks, REM percentage slowly increased, so that at day 27 of treatment REM percentage is only slightly lower than baseline values. Despite this, with discontinuation of desipramine, REM percentage increases to almost 40%. Complete withdrawal with return of baseline REM percentage required almost three weeks. **(B)** Effects of 75 mg clorimpramine on two young men. Initial administration resulted in a complete suppression of REM sleep for several nights. Over the next three weeks, REM percentage slowly increased, so that at day 27 of treatment REM percentage is only slightly lower than baseline values. Despite this, with discontinuation of clorimpramine, REM percentage increased to almost 50%. Complete withdrawal with return of baseline REM percentage required almost three weeks. (Reprinted with permission from Dunleavy DLF, Brezinova V, Oswald I, Maclean AW, Tinker M. Changes during weeks in effects of tricyclic drugs on the human brain. *Brit J Psychiatry.* 1972;120:663–672.)

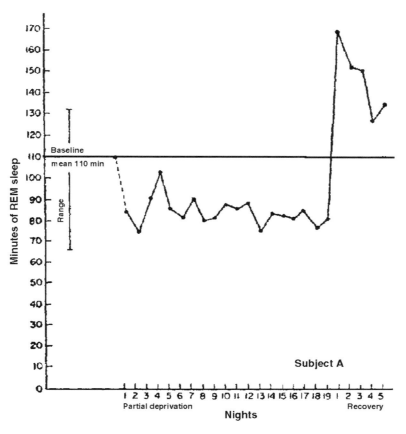

FIGURE 2-4

Effects of partial REM sleep deprivation. Plot of partial REM sleep deprivation and recovery for a single, male, 22–24-year-old subject. Baseline sleep was recorded for 10 consecutive nights. REM sleep was limited to 75% of baseline REM sleep for 19 consecutive nights followed by 5 recovery nights. Total sleep time was 432 min during baseline, 420 min during partial REM deprivation, and 441 min during recovery. REM sleep averaged 110 min (25.5%) baseline, 82 min (19.5%) partial REM deprivation, and 146 min (33.1%) recovery. REM sleep time on the first recovery night was 54% above baseline values. Such data strongly suggests the REM sleep loss is cumulative and loss of a relatively small fraction of REM sleep on a nightly basis over days or weeks contributes to a growing REM sleep debt or REM sleep pressure that continues until allowed to discharge. (Reprinted from *J Psychiat Res*. vol. 4, Dement D, Greenberg S, Klein R. The effect of partial REM deprivation and delayed recovery, 141–152, 1966 with permission of Excerpta Medical Inc.)

Circadian Modulation of Sleep/Wake System (Timing of Sleep)

Sleep and wakefulness typically occur as part of a 24-hour cycle. The measurement of sleep and wakefulness must take into consideration the patient's usual sleep/wake cycle. Failure to schedule the polysomnogram so that the patient can sleep during his or her usual sleep period can result in substantial problems in interpretation.

- Setting a sleep laboratory bedtime and wake time earlier than usual for the patient most often results in
  1. Long sleep latency.
  2. Delayed REM sleep latency (depending on definition).
  3. Reduced total sleep time.
  4. Low sleep efficiency.
  5. Low REM (in minutes and percentage).
- Setting sleep laboratory bedtime and wake time later than usual for the patient most often results in
  1. Short sleep latency.
  2. Short REM sleep latency.
  3. High sleep efficiency.
  4. High REM (in minutes and percentage).
  5. Decreased deep sleep.

These changes occur because many aspects of normal sleep are linked to the circadian rhythm of body temperature. By asking the patient to go to sleep early or late, the sleep specialist is essentially changing the

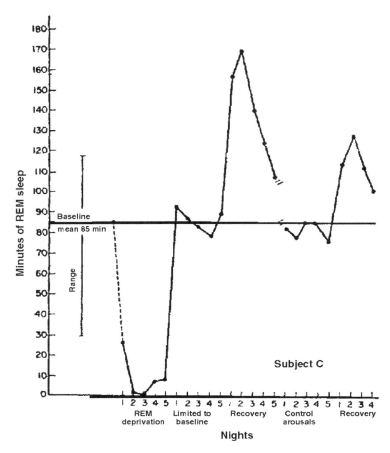

FIGURE 2-5

Total REM sleep deprivation and delayed recovery. Plot of complete REM sleep deprivation, delayed recovery, and full recovery for a single, male, 22–24-year-old subject. Baseline sleep was recorded for 10 consecutive nights. REM sleep was reduced as close to 100% as possible for 5 nights. REM sleep then was allowed to return to the average REM sleep time noted during the 10 baseline nights for 5 nights and to recovery freely for 5 additional nights. In this subject, baseline REM sleep averaged 85 min (19.8%). Complete REM deprivation permitted an average of only 9 min (2.4%) over 5 nights. Limited recovery permitted an average of 84 min (20.6%) over 5 nights. Despite the return to normal quantities and percentages of REM sleep for 5 nights, 142 min (32.3%) was noted during the full recovery period. On the first full night of recovery sleep, REM sleep time was 190 min, or 100% of baseline values. This was equal to or higher than what might be expected after 5 days of complete REM sleep deprivation. These findings strongly suggest that, following REM sleep deprivation, a return to previous normal quantities of REM sleep is insufficient to discharge the REM sleep debt or pressure.

The plot also shows a second study, occurring 2 weeks after the first. In this study, after 10–20 min uninterrupted REM sleep, a patient was awakened an unspecified number of times from REM sleep until baseline levels of REM sleep were present. This was done for 5 days followed by 5 full recovery nights. Average REM sleep time during REM deprivation was 82 min (19.2%) and during recovery, 118 min (26.6%). (Reprinted from *J Psychiat Res.* vol. 4, Dement D, Greenberg S, Klein R. The effect of partial REM deprivation and delayed recovery, 141–152, 1966 with permission of Excerpta Medical Inc.)

relationship between sleep and the circadian rhythm of body temperature. For example, Figure 2-6 shows that short REM sleep latencies are much more likely to occur during the early rising phase of the body temperature, such as usually occurs in the 2–3 hours before the end of a typical sleep period. This may be important not only in interpreting nocturnal sleep studies but in noting the presence of sleep-onset REM periods (SOREMPs) during early naps on the Multiple Sleep Latency Test (MSLT).[15]

The interpreter always should consult the sleep log to determine if the timing of sleep during the polysomnogram is consistent with the usual timing of sleep and wakefulness of the patient at home.

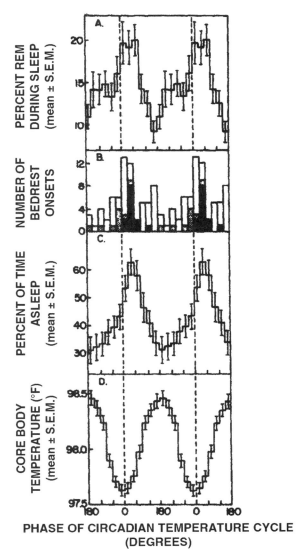

PHASE OF CIRCADIAN TEMPERATURE CYCLE (DEGREES)

FIGURE 2-6

Sleep and circadian temperature. Data from four male subjects living for a total of 94 days on self-selected schedules in an environment free of time cues. The phase of core body temperature can be seen in the bottom plot, D. In plot B, periods of REM sleep that occurred within 10 min of onset of bedrest are in black. Periods of REM sleep that occurred within 30 min of start of bedrest periods are crosshatched. All the shortest REM sleep latencies occurred on the rising part of the temperature curve. (Reprinted with permission from Czeisler CA, Zimmerman JC, Ronda JM, Moore-Ede MC, Weitzman ED. Timing of REM sleep is coupled to the circadian rhythm of body temperature in man. *Sleep.* 1980; (2):329–346.)

3

Evaluating Sleep Stages

Sleep data cannot be interpreted directly from the summary sheets without placing such data within the proper context. The following items always should be considered when interpreting any sleep data:

- Comparison to usual values:
  Workdays or days off?
  What is patient's estimation of sleep quantity and quality at home? In the laboratory?
  Report of bed partner or family.
  Resource: Examine sleep logs/patient history for as many days as possible prior to polysomnogram (PSG).
- Comparison to normative data:
  Compare to age and sex norms.
  Resource: Examine tables of normative data.
- Medication effects (review medication list):
  Any medication sedating or alerting?
  Any medication known to suppress rapid eye movement (REM) or deep sleep?
  Any changes in medication list or dosage in the last 2–4 weeks?
  Alcohol?
  Caffeine?
  Nicotine?
- Sleep/wake schedule (circadian) effects (examine patients' sleep log and history):
  Any recent changes to sleep/wake schedule?
  Shift work?
  On call?
  Recent travel through multiple time zones?
  Naps?
  Recent change in napping behavior?

Was patient scheduled to sleep during usual sleep hours?
Was patient given sufficient time for usual pre-bedtime routines?
Resource: Sleep log and patient questionnaire.
- Effect of sleep disorders: By history or as indicated at other locations in the PSG summary, any documented sleep disorders such as sleep apnea, periodic leg movements that might have caused the patient to awaken and then not be able to return to sleep.
  Resource: Patient history, examination and questionnaire as well as other PSG summary data.
- Technical considerations (unexpected events during the recording night):
  Noise.
  Light.
  Patient complaints.
  Power failure.
  Fire alarms.
  Repeated entry of technicians into the patient room to make adjustments.
  Patient illness, allergies.
  Resources: Technician notes, videotape, patient PM and AM questionnaires.

TOTAL RECORDING TIME

Definition

The total recording time (TRT) is the total amount of time—usually in minutes—during which the patient is in bed with recording equipment activated. Usually from "lights out" (LO) to "lights on" (LON), as noted by the polysomnographic technologist.

General Significance

The amount of time actually spent in bed is one limiting factor of total sleep time and sleep stages. A patient who spends only 3–4 hr in bed cannot reasonably accumulate normal amounts of sleep. Therefore, a low TRT, if selected by the patient, may be of clinical significance and suggest the diagnosis of insufficient sleep. Alternately, it may indicate that the patient spent insufficient time in bed to get an adequate sample of sleep.

Alternative Terms

Time in bed (TIB) differs from TRT in that TIB does not assume that all data have been recorded and are available for analysis.

Possible Explanations for Atypical Total Recording Time

Low TRT may be the result of one or more of these factors:

- Short sleeper by habit or physiology.
- Disturbed by laboratory environment, electrodes, and the like.
- First night effect (FNE).
- Depression or anxiety.
- Sleep/wake schedule disorder.
- Recent intake of alerting medication, such as caffeine or nicotine.
- Recent nap or high total sleep time (TST) on previous night or nights.

High TRT may be the result of one or more of these factors:

- Long sleeper by habit or physiology.
- Rebound sleep following prior restriction of TIB or TST.
- Increased TRT due to anticipatory anxiety about not sleeping.
- Rebound sleep following elimination of a sleep fragmenting process as in first night of successful nasal continuous positive airway pressure (NCPAP) treatment for obstructive sleep apnea (OSA).
- Lack of usual time cues or removal of usual time pressures:
  Took next day off from work.
  No alarm clock.

- Factors that disturb sleep at home not present:
  Reduced noise.
  Darker room.
  No disruption by bed partner (no snoring, poking, tossing, or turning).
  No disruption by children or pets during night.
  No need to wake up to walk dog.
- Work- or marital-related stresses not present.
- Better mattress, pillows, service.
- Felt more secure being monitored all night.
- Could not fall asleep or stay asleep in laboratory and decided to allow more TIB to get enough sleep.
- Recent intake of sedating medications or withdrawal from alerting medications.

Sample Statements

- The total recording time noted in this recording is less than expected for a patient of this age. However, it does confirm the patient's history and suggests a finding of chronic insufficient sleep due to the patient habitually limiting his time in bed.
- The total recording time noted in this recording is less than expected for a patient of this age. The patient noted on her AM questionnaire that she was unable to relax in the laboratory. She specifically noted that the bed was uncomfortable and felt she could not sleep in her usual position. After several hours of fitful sleep, she decided to terminate the recording and leave the sleep laboratory. Therefore, the limited data in this sleep recording may not be sufficient to document the patient's usual sleep patterns.
- The total recording time noted in this recording is far more than expected for a patient of this age and far more than the patient reports usually spending in bed at home. The high TRT and the relatively good sleep quality are likely to be a result of rebound sleep due to partial cumulative sleep deprivation resulting from the patient spending too little time in bed during the workweek. The patient noted on his AM questionnaire that he had taken the day off from work to make sure he slept enough for the sleep study.

TOTAL SLEEP TIME

Definition

The TST is the total amount of sleep time scored during TRT: minutes of stage 1 sleep + stage 2 sleep +

stage 3 sleep + stage 4 sleep + REM sleep—usually in minutes.

General Significance

A low TST may be of clinical significance or indicate that the patient slept an insufficient time due to non-medical, nonphysiological reasons. Low TST may be consistent with a complaint of nonrestorative sleep or daytime sleepiness. A high TST may be the result of either clinical or laboratory factors. High TST may indicate prior sleep deprivation. High levels of sleep fragmentation may result in complaints of nonrestorative sleep, even when an apparently normal TST is present.

Alternative Term

Sleep period may be used instead of TST.

Possible Explanations for Atypical Total Sleep Time

Low TST may result from one or more of the following factors:

- Short sleeper by habit or physiology.
- Reduced by frequent arousals caused by sleep disorders.
- Reduced by difficulty falling asleep.
- Reduced by early morning awakening.
- Reduced by difficulty returning to sleep after awakening.
- Disturbed by laboratory environment, electrodes, and the like.
- Depression or anxiety
- Sleep/wake schedule disorder.
- Recent intake of alerting medication, caffeine, or nicotine.
- Recent nap or high TST on previous night or nights.

High TST may result from one or more of these factors:

- Long sleeper by habit or physiology.
- Arousals following sleep disorders too short to be counted using R&K principles.
- Rebound sleep following prior acute or partial cumulative restriction of TIB or TST.
- Rebound sleep following elimination of a sleep fragmenting process, as in the first night of successful NCPAP treatment for OSA.
- Lack of usual time cues or removal of usual time pressures:
  Took next day off from work.

No alarm clock.
- Factors that disturb sleep at home not present:
  Reduced noise.
  Darker room.
  No disruption by bed partner (no snoring, poking, tossing, or turning).
  No disruption by children or pets during night.
  No need to wake up to walk dog.
- Work, family, or marital related stresses not present.
- Better mattress, pillows, service.
- Felt more secure being monitored all night.
- Recent intake of sedating medications or withdrawal from alerting medications.

Other Considerations

Compare TST on PSG summary with patient estimates on AM questionnaire and with prior sleep history as documented on sleep log data. If summary data is significantly higher than subjective estimate, consider sleep state misperception due to either sleep fragmentation or psychological factors. This suggests that the patient may be sleeping more at home than reported. Sleep state misperception is a common feature of insomnia.[16]

Sample Statements

- The total sleep time noted in this recording is less than expected for a patient of this age. However, it does confirm the patient's history and so suggests a finding of insufficient sleep or short sleeper.
- The total sleep time noted in this recording is far more than expected for a patient of this age and far more than the patient usually reports sleeping at home. Along with the relatively good sleep quality, high TST is suggestive of rebound sleep due to partial cumulative sleep deprivation resulting from the patient restricting time in bed during the workweek.
- The total sleep time noted in this recording is lower than expected for a patient of this age. However, the patient was awakened twice by the sounding of a fire alarm and could not return to sleep for almost 2 hr on each occasion. Therefore, the total sleep time could not be considered typical of the patient's sleep at home, Despite the disruption to the patient's sleep, 4 hr of sleep was recorded, including 30 min of REM sleep. Periodic leg movements in sleep (PLMS) were not present and only mild sleep-disordered breathing occurred in association with the REM sleep.

SLEEP EFFICIENCY

Definition

Sleep efficiency (SE) refers to the percentage of TIB or TRT actually spent in sleep. Typically computed as stage 1 + stage 2 + stage 3 + stage 4 + REM divided by TRT (hrs) × 100.

General Significance

SE gives an overall sense of how well the patient slept but does not distinguish frequent, brief periods of wakefulness from long, sustained periods of wakefulness. A low SE percentage could result from long sleep latency and long sleep offset with otherwise normal quantity and quality of sleep in between. The interpreter always should evaluate sleep efficiency with other sleep parameters to give a better picture of sleep quality.

Possible Explanations for Atypical Sleep Efficiency

Low SE may result from one or more of these factors:

- Short sleeper who remains in bed once awake.
- Sleep disorders
- Anxiety or depression
- Long sleep latency due to first night effect (FNE).
- Long sleep offset period of wakefulness due to depression.
- Recent intake of analeptic medication, caffeine, or nicotine.
- FNE resulting in frequent awakenings.
- Excessive napping or higher than normal TST on prior night.
- Environmental disturbance:
  Noise.
  Light.
  Entry of technician into sleep room.
  Uncomfortable bed.
  Uncomfortable temperature.

High SE may result from one or more of these factors:

- Normal sleeper.
- Rebound sleep.
- Hypnotic or sedative drug effects.
- Periods of wakefulness too short to be scored by the majority of epoch (MOE) rule.

Sample Statements

- The sleep efficiency noted in this recording is lower than expected for a patient of this age. However, almost all the wake time recorded came during a single 3-hr period at the beginning of the recording. Once the patient fell asleep, almost no wake time was noted and good quantities and percentages of deep sleep and REM sleep were present. This strongly suggests that the low sleep efficiency was not characteristic of the patient's usual sleep at home. This sleep pattern could be secondary to difficulty adapting to the sleep laboratory or that the patient's biological best time for sleep onset was 3 hours later than lights out in the laboratory.
- The sleep efficiency noted in this recording is lower than expected for a patient of this age. However, almost all the wake time recorded came during frequent brief periods of wakefulness, rarely exceeding 30 sec, associated with the apneas, hypopneas, or periodic leg movements in sleep. The low sleep efficiency therefore is a marker of severe sleep fragmentation found throughout this recording.
- The 99.5% sleep efficiency noted in this recording is considerably higher than expected for a patient of this age. The presence of a higher than expected percentage of stage 2 sleep, low percentage of deep sleep, and the frequent sleep spindles suggests the high sleep efficiency most likely is secondary to the effects of hypnotic or sedative medication.

See Figure 3-1 for additional examples of sleep-efficiency-related case statements.

TOTAL WAKE TIME

Definition

The total wake time (TWT) is the amount of wake time during TRT/TIB, in minutes. It is the total of all epochs scored as wake using R&K principles.

General Significance

The total amount and percentage gives a general estimation for overall quality of sleep. TWT is the reciprocal of TST. A high TST percentage always is associated with low TWT percentage, and vice versa. However, TWT does not distinguish multiple short periods of wakefulness, consistent with disorders such as sleep apnea, from long sustained periods of wakefulness, consistent with different forms of insomnia or biological rhythm disorders. TWT does not include periods of wakefulness too short to be scored using R&K principles.

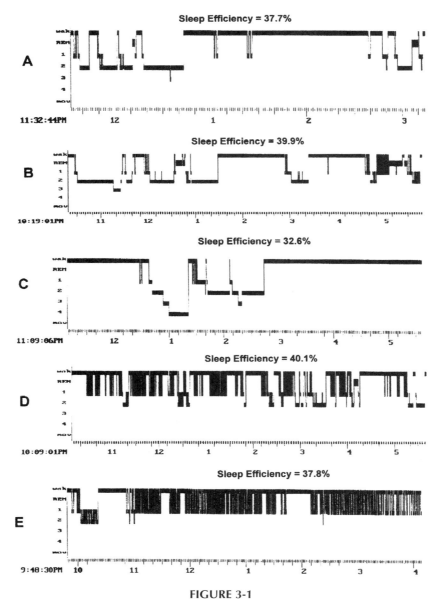

FIGURE 3-1

Sleep-efficiency-related case vignettes. All the sleep histograms in this figure have similar sleep efficiencies, despite being the result of very different types of sleep disturbances. This demonstrates that sleep efficiency—although one of the most easily understood and computed sleep statistics—often is insufficient to describe the quality of sleep. **(A)** Sleep efficiency = 37.7%. The sleep histogram of an 83-year-old woman who presented with a complaint of awakening after 1–3 hr of sleep and experiencing difficulty returning to sleep. Total sleep time was only 83.5 min; total wake time, 138.5 min; and wake after sleep onset and offset, 136 min. Initial period of sustained wakefulness started at 12:45 AM, resulted from a series of arousing periodic leg movements in sleep (APLMS). On the morning questionnaire, the patient described difficulty returning to sleep due to anxiety and rumination. She also reported that this was typical of her sleep at home. The patient fell back to sleep slightly before 3 AM, but on awakening again, insisted that the sleep study be terminated. The final diagnoses were periodic limb movements in sleep and psychophysiological insomnia. **(B)** Sleep efficiency = 39.9%. Sleep histogram of a 57-year-old man during a NCPAP titration night. First sustained period of wakefulness occurred at 1:20 AM, following an increase from 10 cm H_2O to 12.5 cm H_2O. The patient was unable to return to sleep for more than 90 min, although NCPAP pressure was decreased to 0.0 cm H_2O within 5 min. **(C)** Sleep efficiency = 32.6%. Sleep histogram of a 32-year-old man during a diagnostic PSG (DPSG). The patient was referred for evaluation of difficulty falling asleep and daytime fatigue. The final diagnoses were irregular sleep/wake schedule and a sleep disorder associated with an anxiety disorder. **(D)** Sleep efficiency = 40.1%. The sleep histogram from a DPSG of a 48-year-old woman referred for evaluation of obstructive sleep apnea. The overall Respiratory Disturbance Index (RDI) was 65/hr of sleep. Total sleep time was 181.5 min. The sleep histogram shows several periods of wakefulness lasting 10–20 min as well as several periods of stage 2 sleep lasting 5–10 min. Approximately 50% of all epochs scored as wake contained 5–10 sec of scorable stage 1 sleep. **(E)** Sleep efficiency = 37.8%. The sleep histogram of a 58-year-old man evaluated for sleep apnea. RDI = 92/hr. Total sleep time was 143 min, stage 1 was 92% and stage 2, 8%. There are several sustained periods of wakefulness lasting 5–20 min with no sustained periods of stage 2 sleep.

21

Possible Explanations for Atypical Total Wake Time

Low TWT may result from one or more of these factors:

- Normal sleep.
- Rebound sleep.
- Hypnotic or sedative effects of medication.
- Periods of wakefulness too short to be scored by the MOE rule.

High TWT may result from one or more of these factors:

- Sleep disorders.
- FNE.
- Analeptic or activating medication effects.
- Caffeine or nicotine effects.
- Anxiety.
- Depression.
- Environmental disturbance:
  Noise.
  Light.
  Entry of technician into sleep room.
  Uncomfortable bed.
  Uncomfortable temperature.

Sample Statements

- The total wake time noted in this recording is more than expected for a patient of this age. The distribution of wake time in several periods of wakefulness lasting 10–30 min each is consistent with the patient's complaint and suggestive of sleep maintenance insomnia associated with anxiety and racing thoughts.
- The total wake time noted in this recording is less than expected for a patient of this age and far less than the patient reports usually sleeping at home. Additionally, the patient underestimated total sleep time on the AM questionnaire. The patient's high estimate of wake time in the absence of objective confirmation on the PSG suggests that the patient may have difficulty in perceiving sleep when it occurs and actually may be sleeping considerably more than reported by history.

WAKE AFTER SLEEP ONSET

Definition

Wake after sleep onset (WASO) refers to wakefulness occurring after defined sleep onset.

General Significance

This parameter measures wakefulness, excluding the wakefulness occurring before sleep onset. By eliminating wake time occurring before sleep onset, WASO gives a better picture of how much wakefulness occurred during sleep and thus is a better reflection of sleep disruption. This is important, as long sleep latencies are not unusual during PSG due to FNE. The sleep and wakefulness that occurs after sleep onset therefore is more representative of typical sleep at home. Nevertheless, it does not distinguish between multiple, short periods of wakefulness and long, sustained periods of wakefulness.

Possible Explanations for Atypical Wake after Sleep Onset

Low WASO may result from one or more of these factors:

- Normal sleep.
- Rebound sleep.
- Hypnotic or sedative effects of medication.
- Periods of wakefulness too short to be scored by the MOE rule.
- Biological rhythm disturbances, such as delayed sleep phase syndrome, especially if sleep latency was long.

High WASO may result from one or more of these factors:

- Environmental disturbance:
  Noise.
  Light.
  Entry of technician into sleep room.
  Uncomfortable bed.
  Uncomfortable temperature.
- Sleep disorders:
  Sleep apnea.
  PLMS.
  REM behavior disorder (RBD).
  Parasomnias.
  Seizures.
- FNE.
- Analeptic or activating medications effects.
- Alcohol.
- Caffeine or nicotine effects.
- Anxiety.
- Depression.

Sample Statements

- The patient fell asleep almost immediately, but significant quantities of wakefulness were noted during the remainder of the recording. These consisted of seven 15–30 min awakenings, all following external noises. During these periods, the patient appeared restless and told the technical staff he experienced anxiety that interfered with his ability to fall back to sleep.

- After a 2.7 hr sleep latency the patient fell asleep and slept with almost no arousals or wakefulness until awakening after 9 hr in bed. The WASO consisted of only 3 min, suggesting that the quality of sleep was normal once the patient actually fell asleep. This is consistent with a diagnosis of delayed sleep phase syndrome.

WAKE AFTER SLEEP OFFSET

Definition

Wake after sleep offset (WASF) refers to wakefulness that occurs after sleep offset.

General Significance

Long periods of wakefulness following an atypically early AM awakening could be consistent with "an early morning awakening," one of the classic diagnostic signs of depression. This pattern frequently can be found in elderly patients, who may have no difficulty falling asleep but awaken after 3–4 hr of sleep and are unable to return to sleep. Occasionally, patients may remain in bed for long periods after awakening because they are too groggy to get up. Finally, an early awakening with difficulty falling back asleep may be due to FNE and result from suddenly awakening to find oneself in strange surroundings.

Alternative Term

WASF sometimes is called early morning awakening.

Possible Explanations for Atypical Wake after Sleep Offset

Low WASF may result from one or more of these factors:

- Normal sleep.
- Rebound sleep.
- Hypnotic or sedative effects of medication.
- Periods of wakefulness too short to be scored by the MOE rule.

High WASF may result from one or more of these factors:

- Depression.
- Sleep disorders causing nonrestorative sleep or AM grogginess.
- FNE.
- Anxiety.
- Poor laboratory procedures.
- Learned insomnia.
- Environmental disturbance:
  Noise.
  Light.
  Entry of technician into sleep room.
  Uncomfortable bed.
  Uncomfortable temperature.

Sample Statements

- The patient awoke spontaneously after 4 hr of total sleep time and was unable to return to sleep thereafter. During this time she complained of racing thoughts. This pattern was consistent with the patient's usual pattern at home and is suggestive of depression or anxiety.
- The patient was awakened at 3 AM by the night shift technologist, who was making adjustments to dislodged sensors. The patient was unable to return to sleep, thereafter complaining about the loud snoring emanating from the next patient room. The long wake time after sleep offset and short TRT and TST therefore were artifacts of the testing environment and not representative of the patient's usual sleep.

SLEEP LATENCY

Definition

Sleep latency (SL) is the time in minutes from lights out—the official start of either TIB or TRT—to the first epoch scored as sleep. Typically this is to stage 1 sleep, but any sleep stage is acceptable.

Alternative Definitions

Some interpreters believe that stage 1 sleep is only a transitional stage or not "real" physiological sleep. Many interpreters believe sleep onset should be determined by the shift from wakefulness to a less ambiguous stage of sleep. Therefore, some interpreters define sleep latency (sleep onset) as the time from the start of TIB or TRT to the first sleep spindle. Others prefer evidence that sleep has been truly established or that *persistent sleep* is present and so measure it as the time from start of TIB/TRT to the first three consecutive epochs of sleep or first three epochs of stage 2 sleep. More complicated formulas also exist.

General Significance

When *sleep latency* is defined by the requirement for several consecutive epochs of sleep, it may be difficult to apply or be misleading in patients whose sleep is very fragmented due to sleep disorders such as sleep apnea. In severe cases of sleep apnea, for instance, three consecutive epochs of sleep may not occur at any time in the recording, presenting the absurd possibility that sleep latency will not be scored. In a similar vein, significant amounts of stage 1 sleep may accumulate before the first sleep spindle or three consecutive epochs of sleep occur. Should sleep that occurs before official sleep onset be included in TST and other sleep staging parameters? In practice, it often is useful to report sleep latency (sleep onset) in more than one way to provide a more accurate description of sleep onset in a particular patient. For instance, if the sleep latency as defined by the first epoch of sleep is 5.0 min, but sleep latency as defined by the occurrence of first sleep spindle is 45 min, it is likely that a significant period of low-quality sleep or fragmented sleep occurred between the two differently defined sleep onsets.

Alternative Term

SL sometimes is described as the time to sleep onset.

Possible Explanations for Atypical Sleep Latency

Short SL may result from one or more of these factors:

- Normal sleeper.
- Rebound sleep.
- Prior acute or partial cumulative sleep deprivation.
- Hypnotic or sedative effects of medication.
- Alcohol effects.
- Sleep disorders.
- Successful treatment of sleep disorders.
- Environment more conducive to sleep than the home bedroom.

Long SL may result from one or more of these factors:

- Learned insomnia or psychophysiological insomnia.
- Restless legs syndrome.
- Anxiety or depression.
- FNE.

- Sleep/wake schedule disturbance:
  Shift work.
  Jet lag.
  On call.
  Daylight savings time.
  Delayed sleep phase syndrome.
  Retirement.
  Hospitalization.
- Age effects.
- Caffeine, nicotine, alerting medications.
- Environmental disturbance:
  Noise.
  Light.
  Entry of technician into sleep room.
  Uncomfortable bed.
  Uncomfortable temperature.

Sample Statements

- The latency to stage 1 sleep was considerably longer than expected for a patient of this age and much longer than the patient reports usually taking to fall asleep at home. This very long sleep latency is most likely secondary to difficulty adapting to the sleep laboratory.
- The latency to stage 1 sleep was much longer than expected for a patient of this age. A review of the patient's sleep diary showed that the patient recently changed work shift. The time of night the patient actually fell asleep in the sleep laboratory was consistent with the patient's habitual bedtime on the previous shift. The long sleep latency therefore represents a probable failure to phase advance on the new shift and is a symptom of a biological rhythm disorder.
- The latency to stage 1 sleep was much shorter than expected for this patient based on his presenting complaints. Sleep efficiency also was much better than expected at 98%. Stage 2 sleep accounted for slightly more than 70% of total sleep time and frequent sleep spindles were present. The patient noted on his AM questionnaire that he had "borrowed" a tab of triazolam from his wife and taken it 15 min before bedtime. This suggests that the good quantity and quality of sleep was secondary to the effects of medication.

RAPID EYE MOVEMENT LATENCY

Definition

REM latency (REMLAT) is the time from the onset of sleep to the first epoch of REM sleep. This is dependent on the definition of *sleep latency*.

General Significance

Changes in REM sleep latency are thought to be potential biological markers for a variety of disorders. REM sleep latency is very sensitive to the effects of medication, sleep deprivation, and shifts in circadian rhythm.

Alternative Terms

REMLAT sometimes is referred to as *onset of dreaming sleep, D-sleep latency,* or *onset of paradoxical sleep.*

Possible Explanations for Atypical Rapid Eye Movement Latency

Short REM latency may result from one or more of these factors:

- Narcolepsy.
- Sleep apnea.
- Sleep/wake schedule disturbance.
- Withdrawal from REM-sleep-suppressing medications or drugs:
Tricyclic antidepressants.
MAO inhibitors.
Amphetamines.
Barbiturates.
Alcohol.
- Depression.
- Rebound sleep following prior acute or partial cumulative sleep deprivation.
- Sleep laboratory bedtime later than usual bedtime.

Long REM latency may result from one or more of these factors:

- Fragmented non-REM (NREM) sleep prior to first REM period.
- Sleep apnea.
- Periodic leg movements in sleep.
- FNE.
- REM-sleep-suppressing medications (Figure 3-2):
Tricyclic antidepressants.
MAO inhibitors.
Amphetamines.
Barbiturates.
Alcohol.
- Sleep/wake schedule disturbance.
- Sleep laboratory bedtime earlier than usual bedtime at home.

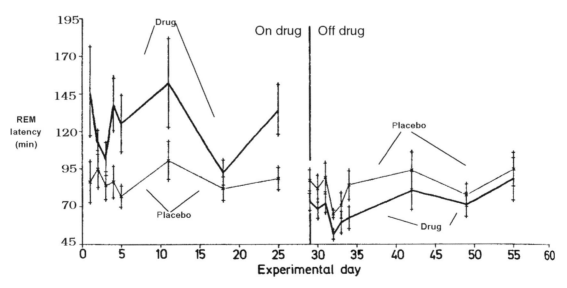

FIGURE 3-2

Effects of amitriptyline administration and withdrawal on REM sleep latency. The figure shows the effects of administration and withdrawal from 50 mg amitriptyline or placebo given nightly to 14 young adults. The administration of tricyclic antidepressants (and other medications that have a REM-sleep-suppressing effect) not only affects REM sleep quantity and percentage but also REM sleep latency. As seen in the figure, administration of amitriptyline delays REM sleep latency while withdrawal results in a shortening of REM latency. REM sleep latency does not return to near normal for more than 2 weeks after withdrawal. (Modified from Hartmann E, Cravens J. The effects of long-term administration of psychotropic drugs on human sleep: III. The effects of amitriptyline. *Psychopharmacologia (Berl).* 1973;33:185–202.)

Additional Considerations

REM sleep can be too short in duration to score. Occasionally, a period of unambiguous REM sleep less than 15 sec in duration may appear with a timing that otherwise would lead to the interpretation of an early REM latency (also called *sleep-onset REM period*, SOREMP). REM sleep does not occur as a "transitional" process following sleep disruption unless the ultradian NREM (non-REM)/REM cycle is in the REM phase. When PSGs are characterized by frequent fragmentation of sleep, a period of REM sleep too short to qualify for scoring under the MOE rule still should be considered for scoring for REM sleep latency. A specific comment should be inserted that, although the brief appearance of REM sleep was not scorable by the R&K MOE rules, it is consistent with the diagnosis of depression or narcolepsy.

Sample Statements

- Rapid eye movement sleep typically occurs 90–120 min after sleep onset. A REM sleep latency of 31 min, noted in this recording, is shorter than expected. REM sleep latencies in this range previously have been reported to be associated with major affective disorders, circadian rhythm disorders, recent discontinuation of REM-sleep-suppressing medication, recent elimination of REM-sleep-fragmenting processes, or relief of recent acute or cumulative partial sleep deprivation.
- Rapid eye movement sleep typically occurs 90–120 minutes after sleep onset. A REM sleep latency of 325 min, noted in this recording, is much longer than expected. The delay of REM sleep latency most likely is due to the effects of antidepressant medication or possibly the alcohol in the three beers the patient noted drinking just before arriving at the sleep laboratory.

STAGE 1 SLEEP

Definition

As defined in R&K, sleep that typically occurs during the transition from wakefulness to sleep of any stage. Stage 1 (S1) sleep generally follows wake and is followed by stage 2 sleep but may occur when stage 2, 3, 4, or REM sleep is disrupted.

General Significance

As S1 is associated with the transition from wakefulness, it is a good measure of how often such transitions from

wakefulness occur. This assumes that S1 lasts long enough to be scored using the standard R&K MOE rules. The quantity and percentage of S1 sleep often are good measures of sleep quality and continuity. The quantity of S1 sleep often directly relates to daytime alertness and the subjective refreshing quality of the sleep.

Alternative Terms

S1 sleep may be called *light sleep* or *transitional sleep*.

Possible Explanations for Atypical Stage 1 Sleep

Low S1 sleep may result from one or more of these factors:

- Rebound sleep (check other sleep stages for high quantity and percentage).
- Hypnotic or sedative effect of medication.
- Normal sleeper.
- Absence of usual environmental disruptions.
- Age effects.
- Reverse FNE.

High S1 sleep may result from one or more of these factors:

- Frequent arousals caused by sleep disorders:
  Sleep apnea.
  Periodic leg movements in sleep.
  Snoring.
- First night effect.
- Drug withdrawal.
- Rare or poorly formed sleep spindles leading to underscoring of stage 2.
- Age effects.
- Environmental disturbances:
  Noise.
  Light.
  Bed.
  Room temperature.
  Disruption by technical staff.

Additional Comments and Considerations

Down and Dirty Estimates of Sleep Fragmentation
The quantity and percentage of S1 sleep is at best an estimate of the degree of sleep fragmentation. Only periods of S1 lasting long enough to qualify under the MOE rule are scored. Therefore, periods of S1 that do not qualify are not included, reducing the apparent amount of sleep fragmentation (Figure 3-3).

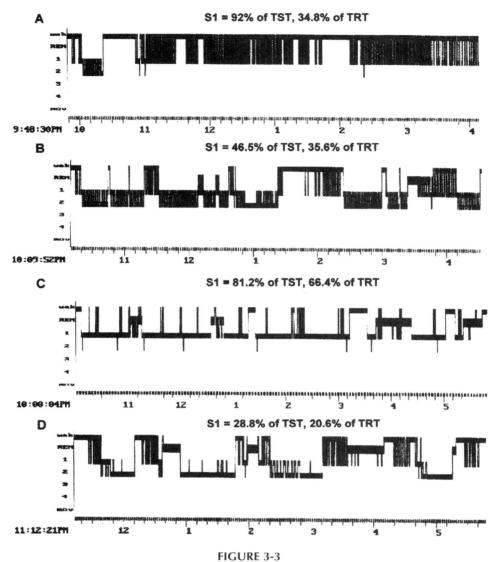

FIGURE 3-3

Stage 1 sleep. The four sleep histograms **(A–D)** appear to be quite different but are all associated with a finding of severe obstructive sleep apnea. The respiratory findings range from a total of 736 apneas or hypopneas in plot A to 433 apneas or hypopneas in plot D. Although the final interpretation and diagnosis does not differ for these four cases, they differ significantly in terms of the composition of sleep stages. Their differences are entirely secondary to the duration of stage 1 sleep and wake time associated with each apnea or hypopnea. The duration of stage 1 sleep and wake time, in turn, are dependent on the duration of apneas or hypopneas and on how quickly characteristics of stage 2 sleep or REM sleep appear on return to sleep following termination of apneas or hypopneas. **(A)** The average duration of apneas and hypopneas was 14 sec. The majority of epochs scored consisted of slightly more than 15 sec of wakefulness and slightly less than 15 sec of stage 1 sleep. After the first 30 min recording time, during which some stage 2 was noted, the longest period of sleep was limited to the duration of the longest apnea or hypopnea. Additionally, during the 14–16 sec of sleep typically noted, sleep spindles did not appear rapidly enough for stage 2 to be scored under the R&K MOE rules. **(B)** The sleep in this plot differs from plot A only in that arousals from sleep were relatively short, averaging <10 sec, and sleep spindles often appeared within 15 sec of the return of sleep. This, in turn, may have been because the average duration of apneas and hypopneas was 28 sec. As a result stage 2 was 46.3%, although 540 apneas and hypopneas appeared repetitively during the recording. **(C)** The profile of sleep disordered breathing here is almost identical to plot B. The sleep in plot C differs from B only in that sleep spindles did not appear rapidly following a return to sleep. This was sufficient to increase S1 sleep to 81.2% of TST and reduce S2 sleep to <3% of TST. **(D)** The profile of sleep disordered breathing in plot D is almost identical to plots B and C. However, the sleep in plot D differs from B and C in that sleep spindles appeared within 5 sec of return to sleep, giving the appearance of continuous stage 2 sleep during periods when apneas and hypopneas appear repetitively.

State Shifts

An alternative way to estimate the degree of sleep fragmentation is to examine the scoring sheets and determine how many times the sleep stage changed. S1 sleep, even if it is too short to be scored, frequently results in a change of sleep stage, even if that is from stage 3 to stage 2.

Respiratory Disturbance Index

The respiratory disturbance index (RDI) often is a good estimate of sleep fragmentation, as almost all apneas and hypopneas are associated with arousal or awakening, especially in patients with moderate and severe sleep apnea.

Periodic Leg Movements in Sleep Index

The PLMS index can be used in the same way, if most PLMS are associated with arousal. The PLMS index should be used as an estimate of sleep fragmentation with some caution, as PLMS-associated arousal often is shorter in duration than OSA-related arousal.

T-Sleep

An alternate method of scoring sleep for PSGs with high levels of sleep fragmentation has been proposed by McGregor and colleagues.[17]

Sample Statements

- The quantity and percentage of stage 1 sleep noted in this recording was well in excess of that expected for a patient of this age. Stage 1 sleep occurred in brief periods following the appearance of apneas, hypopneas, or periodic leg movements and so is an indicator of the overall severe fragmentation of sleep noted in this recording.
- The quantity and percentage of stage 1 sleep noted in this recording was well in excess of that expected for a patient of this age. Stage 1 sleep was scored in extended periods often exceeding 10 min. As stage 1 sleep is a transitional stage of sleep, bridging the gap between wakefulness and sleep, it rarely persists for such lengthy periods of time without a recurring source of arousal. As the quantity and percentage of stage 2 sleep also was considerably less than expected, it seems more likely that these periods of apparent stage 1 sleep actually are stage 2 sleep with infrequent and poorly formed sleep spindles, which would be consistent with the patient's older age.

- The quantity and percentage of stage 1 sleep noted in this recording were higher than expected for a patient of this age. Stage 1 sleep was scored in extended periods, often exceeding 10 min. The histogram of the sleep staging does not properly represent the repetitive, alternating brief periods of wakefulness and slightly longer periods of stage 1 sleep that actually occurred during these periods. An arousal index of 67.5/hr of sleep is more representative of the severe sleep fragmentation noted.

STAGE 2 SLEEP

Definition

Stage 2 (S2) sleep, as defined by R&K, is an intermediate stage of NREM sleep characterized by sleep spindles and K complexes. Delta EEG (electroencephalogram) activity may be present but must occupy less than 20% of the epoch.

General Significance

S2 sleep usually constitutes the largest percentage of total sleep time.

Alternative Terms

Spindle or *sigma sleep* and *intermediate sleep* are terms also used to refer to S2 sleep.

Possible Explanations for Atypical Stage 2 Sleep

Low S2 sleep may result from one or more of these factors:

- Poor spindle activity leads to underscoring.
- Sleep apnea.
- High levels of sleep fragmentation do not permit sufficient time for stage 2 to be established.
- Rebound of REM or slow-wave sleep (SWS).
- Restricted sleep schedule.

High S2 sleep may result from one or more of these factors:

- Medication effect reduces delta sleep activity.
- Medication effect increases spindle activity, such as with benzodiazepines.
- Reduced stage 3 and 4 sleep.
- Age-related changes.

Additional Comments and Considerations

Delta-Frequency Electroencephalogram Activity and Sleep Staging

The R&K definition of *stage 2 sleep* permits the presence of up to 19% delta activity in the scored epoch. In some individuals, considerable quantities of delta activity can be accumulated without ever exceeding the 20% delta activity threshold that triggers the scoring of stage 3 and 4 sleep, the traditional stages of deep sleep. If the sleep record contains quantities of stage 2 delta EEG activity but little or no scored stage 3 and 4 activity, this should be commented on in the interpretation. Otherwise, the erroneous impression of no delta EEG or deep sleep may be given.

K Complexes

The K complex is a common feature of stage 2 sleep. The K complex is one of the first features described when sleep was studied by relatively primitive EEG machines in the late 1930s. It was described then as a "disturbance complex." K complexes most often are thought to characterize arousal during sleep although the source of the arousal is not always evident. For this reason, many K complexes are labeled *spontaneous*, indicating the source is thought to be endogenous activity in the brain or elsewhere. Other K complexes are labeled *evoked*, as they clearly are secondary to external processes.[18] A small literature suggests that spontaneous K complexes are linked to the R wave of the ECG and may be influenced by cardiopulmonary activity.[19] Other K complexes are directly secondary to the arousing effects of sleep-disordered breathing, periodic leg movements in sleep (PLMS), or other things that go bump in the night. These sometimes are labeled *K-alpha complexes*, as alpha EEG activity, characteristic of arousal, immediately follows the K complex. Although, R&K state that both types of K complexes may be used to score stage 2 sleep, scoring of stage 2 sleep following K-alpha complexes may lead to an increase in stage 2 sleep and a reduction in highly significant arousals from sleep (Figure 3-4).

Sleep Spindles

The sleep spindle or sigma waveform is a defining characteristic of stage 2 sleep, according to R&K. The sleep spindle consists of a brief burst of 12–14 Hz activity lasting at least 0.5 sec and rarely longer than 1 sec (Figure 3-5). Sleep spindles generally are considered to represent inhibitory activity in the brain.[20] Central nervous system (CNS) depressant medications, such as benzodiazepines, often result in an increase in the frequency of spindles (Figure 3-6), and spindle rates decline in old age. High rates of spindle activity may indicate the presence of benzodiazepines, even when not reported or even denied by the patient. See Table 3-1 for a selected list of spindle rates in different age groups and the effects of medication.

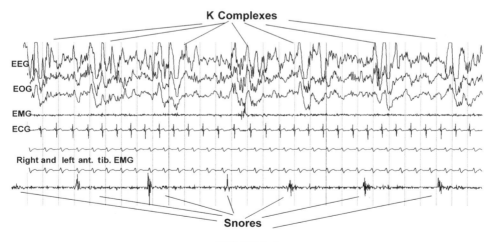

FIGURE 3-4

Evoked K complexes and snores. A 30 sec epoch from the sleep recording of a 45-year-old woman who presented with complaints of loud snoring, nonrestorative sleep, and daytime fatigue. The epoch shows a K complex occurring every 5 sec. The K complex is preceded each time by a snore. Spontaneous K complexes are not periodic, while snoring and sleep-disordered breathing are periodic. Therefore, these K complexes are signs of arousal. This epoch originally was scored as stage 3 sleep. The final diagnosis was upper airway resistance syndrome.

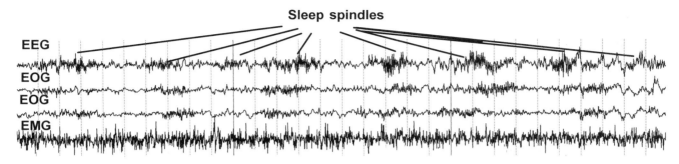

FIGURE 3-5

Frequent sleep spindles. A 30 sec epoch of the diagnostic sleep recording of a 25-year-old man who presented with complaints of difficulty falling asleep and frequent awakenings from sleep. In NREM sleep, 16 sleep spindles/min occurred, more than double the expected rate. An examination of the patient's presleep questionnaire noted no hypnotic or sedative medications known to increase the sleep spindle rate. However, during the follow-up office visit the patient admitted to taking an 1 mg of clonazepam for the two nights prior to the PSG, due to "nervousness" and fear that he would be unable to fall asleep in the sleep laboratory.

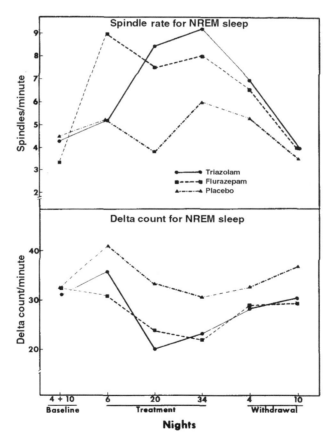

FIGURE 3-6

Drug effects on sleep spindle rates and delta EEG waveform counts. The two plots show sleep spindle rate/min and delta count/min during baseline, treatment, and withdrawal from a short-acting benzodiazepine (triazolam) and a long-acting benzodiazepine (flurazepam). Subjects were 21 diagnosed insomniacs with a mean age of 43 ± 12.7, 17 women and 4 men. Sleep spindles (11.75–15.0 Hz) and delta half waves (0.5–2.0 Hz) were identified with an automatic detector (Smith phasic EEG detector). (Reprinted from *EEG Clin Neurophysiol.* vol. 55, Johnson LC, Spinweber CL, Seidel WF, Dement WC. Sleep spindle and delta changes during chronic use of a short-acting and a long-acting benzodiazepine hypnotic, 662–667, 1983 with permission of Excerpta Medical Inc.)

TABLE 3-1
Sleep Spindle Rates (per minute)

Mean Spindles/ Min	Standard Deviation	Associated Findings and Consequences	Reference
12.2		30 mg flurazepam for 1 night in normals (age 22 yr), increase from 6.9 on baseline	21
8.8	3.0	Insomniacs mean age 43 ± 12.7 yr after 6 days of treatment with flurazepam with dosage unknown	22
8.2	3.2	Insomniacs mean age 43 ± 12.7 yr after 20–34 days of treatment with triazolam with dosage unknown	22
7.8	2.2	Insomniacs mean age 43 ± 12.7 yr after 20–34 days of treatment with flurazepam with dosage unknown	22
7.1		30 mg diphenhydramine for 1 night in normals (age 22 yr)	21
6.9	4.8	Insomniacs mean age 43 ± 12.7 yr after 4 days' withdrawal from triazolam with dosage unknown	22
6.8		45 mg flurazepam for 1 night in young normal adults (mean 25 yr)	23
6.5	3.2	Insomniacs mean age 43 ± 12.7 yr after 4 days' withdrawal from flurazepam with dosage unknown	22
6.3		240 mg phenobarbital for 1 night in young normal adults (mean age 25 yr)	23
6.2		8 mg haloperidol for 1 night in young normal adults (mean age 25 yr)	23
5.7		10 grams L-tryptophan for 1 night in young normal adults (mean age 25 yr)	23
5.2	0.82	Insomniacs mean age 43 ± 12.7 yr after 6 days of treatment with triazolam dosage unknown	22
4.3	2.2	Insomniacs mean age 43 ± 12.7 yr	22
4.0	2.3	Insomniacs mean age 43 ± 12.7 yr after 10 days' withdrawal from triazolam with dosage unknown	22
4.0	1.8	Insomniacs mean age 43 ± 12.7 yr after 10 days' withdrawal from flurazepam with dosage unknown	22
3.5		Normal men mean age 24.8 yr (visual analysis)	24
2.7		Normal men mean age 53.6 yr (visual analysis)	24
0.6		Normal men mean age 72.6 yr (visual analysis)	24

Note: Unless labeled all analyzes done with automatic frequency analyzer.

Sample Statements

- As noted in the summary sleep parameters, deep or slow wave sleep (stages 3 and 4) meeting the usual sleep stage scoring amplitude requirements was not noted in this recording. However, considerable delta frequency EEG activity with lower amplitude nevertheless was present during stage 2 sleep.
- The percentage of stage 2 sleep was higher than expected for a patient of this age. Stage 2 sleep additionally was characterized by a higher number of sleep spindles per minute than expected as well as the intrusion of faster frequency alpha EEG waves and beta frequency EEG waves. This is likely to have resulted from the effects of the lorazepam taken hs by the patient.

STAGE 3 SLEEP

Definition

As defined in R&K, stage 3 (S3) sleep is relatively deep sleep characterized by high amplitude delta EEG waves that occupy 20–50% of the scoring epoch.

General Significance

A high percentage of S3 sleep suggests that a significant percentage of the scored epochs are characterized by delta EEG activity. However, stage 3 is an arbitrary category with no specific clinical correlates. It should be interpreted along with stage 4 sleep and any delta activity occurring during stage 2 sleep.

Alternative Terms

S3 sleep also is called *delta sleep*, *slow-wave sleep (SWS)*, and *deep sleep*.

Possible Explanations for Atypical Stage 3 Sleep

Low S3 sleep may result from one or more of these factors:

- Sleep fragmented by sleep disorders:
  Sleep apnea.
  Periodic leg movements in sleep.
  Night terrors, sleep walking, sleep talking, confusional arousals.
- Medication effects, such as from benzodiazepines, tricyclic antidepressants (TCA), or barbiturates.
- Age.
- FNE.
- Environmental disruption:
  Noise.
  Light.
  Uncomfortable mattress.
  Technician entry into sleep room.

High S3 sleep may result from one or more of these factors:

- Rebound sleep, following the end of partial or total sleep deprivation or elimination of a sleep fragmenting process, such as NCPAP or sleep apnea.
- Successful pharmacotherapy of PLMS.
- Developmental immaturity.

Additional Comments and Considerations

Stage 3 versus Stage 4 Sleep
Traditional R&K scoring requires that S3 and S4 sleep be scored separately. However, the separation of these two stages reflects only the relative quantity of delta frequency EEG activity in a particular epoch. There is no known clinical significance to S3 versus S4 sleep, and in practice they typically are combined to provide a general estimate of SWS or deep sleep.

The Effect of Different Epoch Duration (Chart Speed) on Stage 2, Stage 3, and Stage 4 Sleep Scoring
The American Academy of Sleep Medicine and R&K standards permit scoring using 20 or 30 sec epochs. When using a 20 sec epoch, only 10 sec of delta EEG activity is necessary for the majority of the epoch and a stage 4 score, as opposed to 15 sec of delta EEG activity with a 30 sec epoch. Therefore, the use of 20 sec epochs may increase the percentage of stage 3 and 4 sleep compared to the use of 30 sec epochs.

Sample Statements

- The quantity and percentage of deep sleep (stages 3 and 4) noted in this recording are higher than expected for a patient of this age. The high quantity and percentage of deep sleep is most consistent with rebound sleep, following a period of either acute, total sleep deprivation or chronic, cumulative, partial sleep deprivation. When the patient is deprived of deep sleep it is potentiated and, when permitted to appear, will rebound in quantities higher than normal. The deep sleep rebound noted may have occurred because of changes in the patients sleep/wake schedule or because sleeping in the sleep laboratory excluded certain elements of the patient's usual sleep environment that are disruptive to sleep.
- The substantial increase in deep sleep (stages 3 and 4) seen with administration of NCPAP in this recording is consistent with deep sleep rebound. Deep sleep rebound occurs when a sleep-fragmenting process, such as apneas or hypopneas, is eliminated. Typically, deep sleep increases above normal quantities for several days and thereafter returns to normal. A deep sleep rebound is considered an excellent sign of effective NCPAP treatment.
- The quantity and quality of deep sleep (stages 3 and 4) noted in this recording are lower than expected for a patient of this age. It is likely that the decrease in deep sleep and the related increase in intermediate stage 2 sleep and sleep spindle rates per minute are related to the effects of the flurazepam. Many benzodiazepines decrease the amplitude of delta frequency EEG waves characteristic of deep sleep and increase the number of sleep spindles characteristic of stage 2 sleep.

STAGE 4 SLEEP

Definition

As defined in R&K, stage 4 (S4) sleep is a stage of deep sleep characterized by high-amplitude delta EEG waves occupying >50% of the scored epoch.

General Significance

Stage 4 sleep is a stage of deep sleep with a high arousal threshold.

Alternative Terms

S4 sleep also is called *delta sleep*, *slow-wave sleep*, and *deep sleep*.

Possible Explanations for Atypical Stage 4 Sleep

Low S4 sleep may result from one or more of these factors:

- Sleep fragmented by sleep disorders:
  Sleep apnea.
  Periodic leg movements in sleep.
  Night terrors, sleep walking, sleep talking, confusional arousals.
- Medication effects, such as from benzodiazepines or TCA.
- Age.
- FNE.
- Delta EEG activity that lacks required amplitude.
- Environmental disruption:
  Noise.
  Light.
  Uncomfortable mattress.
  Technician entry into sleep room.

High S4 sleep may result from one or more of these factors:

- Rebound sleep, as from end of partial or total sleep deprivation.
- End of sleep/wake schedule disturbance:
  Recovery from jet lag.
  Recovery from shift work.
  Recovery from on-call.
- Elimination of a sleep fragmenting process, such as NCPAP of sleep apnea or pharmacotherapy of PLMS.
- Extension of TRT and TST.
- Medication effects.
- Developmental immaturity.

Additional Comments and Considerations

Stage 3 versus Stage 4

Traditional R&K scoring requires that S3 and S4 sleep be scored separately. However, the separation of these two stages reflects only the relative quantity of delta frequency EEG activity in a particular epoch. There is no known clinical significance to S3 versus S4 sleep, and in practice they typically are combined to provide an estimate of SWS or deep sleep.

The Effect of Different Epoch Duration (Chart Speed) on Stage 2, Stage 3, and Stage 4 Sleep Scoring

American Academy of Sleep Medicine and R&K standards permit scoring using 20 or 30 sec epochs. When using a 20 sec epoch, only 10 sec of delta EEG activity is necessary for the majority of the epoch and a stage 4 score, as opposed to 15 sec of delta EEG activity with a 30 sec epoch. Therefore, use of 20 sec epochs may increase percentage of stage 3 and 4 sleep compared to use of 30 sec epochs.

Sample Statements

- The quantity and percentage of deep sleep (stages 3 and 4) noted in this recording is higher than expected for a patient of this age. A high quantity and percentage of deep sleep is most consistent with rebound sleep following a period of either acute total sleep deprivation or chronic, cumulative, partial sleep deprivation. When the patient is deprived of deep sleep, deep sleep rebound is potentiated and, when permitted, occurs. The deep rebound noted may have occurred because of changes in the patient's sleep/wake schedule or because sleeping in the sleep laboratory excluded certain elements of the patient's usual sleep environment that are disruptive to sleep.
- The substantial increases in deep sleep (stages 3 and 4) seen with administration of NCPAP in this recording are consistent with deep sleep rebound. Deep sleep rebound occurs when a sleep-fragmenting process, such as apneas or hypopneas, is eliminated. Typically, deep sleep increases to a quantity that is more than expected for a normal patient of this age for several days and thereafter returns to normal. A deep sleep rebound is considered an excellent sign of effective NCPAP treatment.
- The quantity and quality of deep sleep (stages 3 and 4) noted in this recording are lower than expected for a patient of this age. It is likely that the decrease in deep sleep and the related increase in intermediate stage 2 sleep are related to the effects of the flurazepam taken by the patient for the last two months. Some benzodiazepines decrease the amplitude and number of delta frequency EEG waves characteristic of deep sleep and increase the number of sleep spindles characteristic of stage 2 sleep.

See Figure 3-7 for additional examples of slow-wave-sleep-related case statements.

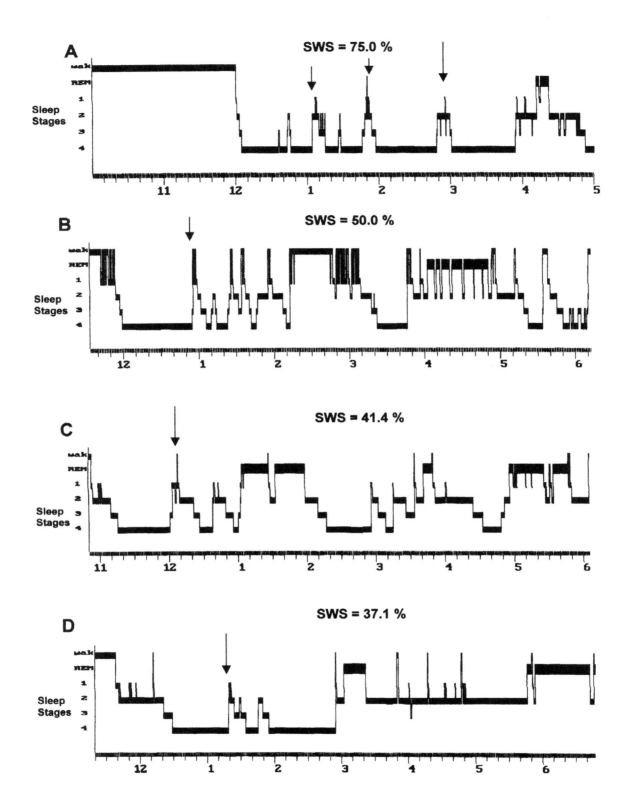

◄ FIGURE 3-7

Slow-wave-sleep-related case vignettes. **(A)** The sleep histogram from the DPSG of a 75-year-old white woman. This patient had been admitted to the inpatient medical service of the hospital for complaints of shortness of breath and fatigue. On admission, the nursing staff noted snoring and apparent apneas. After her 12th day as an inpatient, she had a diagnostic polysomnogram in the sleep disorder center laboratory. A total of 225 min of SWS was noted with only 1.8% stage 1 sleep and 3.3% REM sleep. She noted on her morning questionnaire that she had slept much better than usual in the sleep laboratory and stated that she had been "barely" sleeping while in the hospital. Interpretation of these data assumed this to be an extreme example of SWS rebound following significant sleep deprivation as a hospital patient. Further support for the role of the hospital as a sleep-disturbing environment can be seen in her 120 min sleep latency. According to the patient, she was accustomed to going to sleep before 10 PM prior to entering the hospital. Therefore, the sleep onset at midnight may represent a circadian phase delay that may occur when normal time cues are absent. Despite the report of snoring and witnessed apneas on the inpatient service, only 25 hypopneas (RDI of 4/hr) were noted. As SWS is known to suppress the occurrence of sleep-disordered breathing, the presence of such a large quantity of deep sleep may have invalidated the attempt to diagnose sleep apnea. This hypothesis was supported when she returned for a repeat DPSG two months after discharge from the hospital. A total of only 45 min (12%) SWS and an RDI of 19/hr were noted. Arrows indicate expected timing of REM sleep although only a single epoch is noted at the second arrow from the left. **(B)** The sleep histogram during NCPAP treatment trial for a 44-year-old white woman, 5'4", 220 lbs. Previous DPSG was consistent with severe OSA. Findings included 733 obstructive apneas and hypopneas for an RDI of 133 per hour of sleep. Apneas and hypopneas averaged 13–16 sec in duration. Sleep was severely fragmented for most of the diagnostic recording but included 42 min stage 3 and 4 sleep and 39 min REM sleep. In the NCPAP treatment trial recording, a pressure of 10 cm H_2O was found to be optimal, resulting in a reduction in the RDI to 4.5/hr of sleep. Stage 3 and 4 sleep accounted for 162.5 min, or 50%, total sleep time. REM sleep accounted for 41 min, no different from the DPSG. Therefore, as noted in Figure 3-8, plot A, where REM sleep occupied 63% to total sleep time following initial NCPAP administration, it could not be predicted from the diagnostic sleep study whether SWS would rebound first. However, any type of rebound sleep with NCPAP administration should be considered a positive sign of treatment success. **(C)** The sleep histogram of the DPSG for a 25-year-old male, medical intern referred for evaluation of excessive daytime sleepiness. The patient's sleep log showed only 2 hr of sleep on the nights prior to the recording due to a busy on-call schedule, suggesting significant partial cumulative sleep deprivation as well as a probable biological rhythm disturbance. Patient noted on the morning questionnaire that his sleep in the sleep laboratory was the longest period he had slept in three weeks. It therefore is suggestive of rebound slow wave sleep and provides diagnostic support for a diagnosis of insufficient sleep and shift work schedule disorder. **(D)** The sleep histogram from the DPSG for a 53-year-old woman who was referred for evaluation of difficulty falling and staying asleep. A total of 145 min of stage 3 and 4 sleep, or 37.1%, SWS sleep were noted. This was in excess of the expected SWS percentage for a woman of this age. The DPSG was negative for sleep apnea and periodic leg movements in sleep. The sleep log showed no recent changes in sleep/wake schedule or medication. However, the patient had noted on her morning questionnaire that she had "slept much better than usual" and awakened "feeling much more alert than usual." She specifically noted that the sleep laboratory room was much quieter and darker than her home bedroom and that she felt more secure being monitored in the hospital. She further noted she lived close to a noisy intersection and that her husband snored loudly. In this case, the sleep laboratory provided a rare night away from an environment not conducive for good-quality sleep and suggested the diagnosis of an environmental sleep disorder.

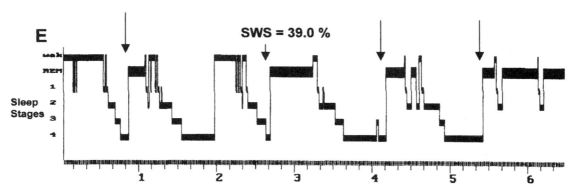

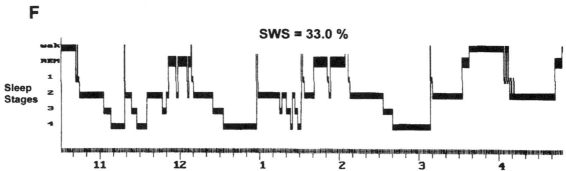

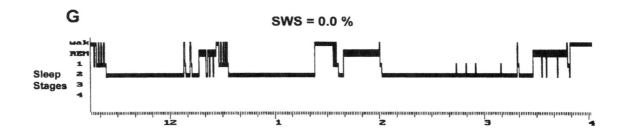

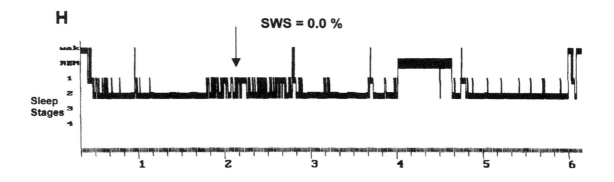

◄ **FIGURE 3-7** *continued*

(E) The sleep histogram of the initial NCPAP treatment trial of a 37-year-old man who previously had been diagnosed with severe obstructive sleep apnea. The DPSG had shown 524 obstructive apneas and hypopneas for an RDI of 125.5/hr of sleep. No deep sleep was noted and only 25 min, or 10%, REM sleep. Stage 1 sleep accounted for 41% of total sleep time. With administration of NCPAP, the RDI was reduced to 8.5/hr; SWS increased to 117.5 min, or 33%; and REM sleep increased to 126.5 min, or 39%. Both SWS and REM sleep rebounded to a similar degree at the expense of stage 1 sleep, now only 18 min, or 5.6%, of TST and stage 2 sleep, now 48 min, or 18%, of TST. Arrows indicate repeated direct shifts from stage 4 sleep to REM sleep with no intervening stage 2 or 3 sleep continued throughout the recording. These shifts strongly suggest substantial pressure for both SWS and REM sleep. **(F)** The sleep histogram from the DPSG of a 16-year-old male high school student who was referred for evaluation due to repeated episodes of dozing in class. A total of 109 min stage 3 and 4 sleep, or 33% SWS, were noted before polysomnographic recording was terminated at the request of the patient. Although, a 33% SWS is slightly higher than expected for a 16 year old, it is not as high as noted in the other cases presented in this figure. The appearance of a third SWS cycle with stage 4 sleep is unusual, as is the lower than expected percentage of REM sleep—14%. Based on this finding plus a sleep log, a final diagnosis of insufficient sleep due to sleep/wake schedule disturbance was made. **(G)** The sleep histogram from the diagnostic PSG of a 47-year-old woman who presented with a 10-year complaint of difficulty falling asleep. Patient had been taking 30 mg flurazepam nightly since the onset of the complaint. The sleep EEG was characterized by frequent sleep spindles and the absence of delta frequency activity that met the 75 μV amplitude criterion. Complete absence of SWS therefore is likely a function of the medication effects. **(H)** The sleep histogram from a diagnostic polysomnogram of a 74-year-old man who presented with a complaint of snoring and frequent awakenings from sleep. Patient medications included 15 mg temazepam hs. The sleep histogram shows complete absence of SWS, plus some evidence of sleep apnea. Arrow indicates a sustained period during which sleep is highly fragmented, in this case by hypopneas while in the supine position. The complete absence of SWS is likely secondary to a combination of the expected age-related changes, benzodiazepines, and sleep disruption by apneas.

RAPID EYE MOVEMENT SLEEP

Definition

As defined in R&K, REM sleep is one of two general states of sleep characterized by low voltage/fast frequency EEG, muscle atonia, and rapid eye movements. Dreaming usually is associated with this state.

General Significance

Although the exact function of REM sleep is uncertain, fragmentation or deprivation of it can result in decreased daytime alertness. Also, REM sleep is associated with more-frequent and longer-duration apneas and hypopneas, as well more severe hypoxia. REM sleep typically suppresses periodic leg movements in sleep.

Alternative Terms

Other terms for REM sleep are *paradoxical sleep*, *D-sleep*, and *dreaming sleep*.

Possible Explanations for Atypical Rapid Eye Movement Sleep

Low REM sleep may result from one or more of these factors:

- Fragmenting effects of sleep disorders:
  Sleep apnea.
  REM behavior disorder.
  Nightmares.
- Effects of REM-sleep-suppressing medication, such as
  Amphetamines.
  Barbiturates.
  TCAs.
  MAO inhibitors.
  Anticholinergics.
  Alcohol.
- Age.
- Sleep/wake schedule disorder.
- Environmental disruption:
  Noise.
  Light.
  Uncomfortable mattress.
  Technician entry into sleep room.

High REM sleep may result from one or more of these factors:

- Rebound following a period of REM sleep deprivation caused by

Successful treatment of sleep-fragmenting disorder.
Discontinuation of REM-sleep-suppressing medication or alcohol.
Recent change in sleep/wake schedule.
End of period of acute or partial cumulative sleep deprivation.
- Age.

Additional Comments and Considerations

Occasionally a period of unambiguous REM sleep less than 15 sec may be present. REM sleep does not occur as a "transitional" process following sleep disruption unless the ultradian NREM/REM cycle is in the REM phase. Obstructive sleep apnea occurs more frequently during REM sleep and may cause arousal, ending REM sleep only seconds after it has begun. In PSGs characterized by frequent fragmentation of sleep due to sleep apnea or frequent arousal from REM sleep, as is often seen in narcolepsy, a period of REM sleep may be too short to qualify for scoring under the majority of the epoch rule. For example, in the case of REM-sleep-exacerbated hypoxia, a comment should be made that, even though the MOE rule prevented the scoring of REM sleep, the hypoxia was likely to be secondary to the effects of REM sleep.

Sample Statements

- The quantity and percentage of REM sleep in this recording is higher than expected for a patient of this age and most consistent with a REM sleep rebound. A REM sleep rebound could occur following discontinuation of a REM-sleep-suppressing medication (e.g., TCAs, MAO inhibitors, alcohol), following elimination of REM-sleep-fragmenting events (e.g., apneas, hypopneas), recent acute or chronic partial sleep deprivation, or a change in usual sleep/wake schedule.
- The substantial increase in REM sleep noted with the administration of NCPAP is consistent with REM sleep rebound. REM sleep rebound occurs when a REM sleep fragmentation caused by apneas, hypopneas, or snoring is eliminated. This permits the return of uninterrupted REM sleep. However, REM sleep typically returns with quantities that are higher than expected for several days and then reverts to normal. A REM sleep rebound is considered an excellent sign of successful NCPAP treatment.
- The quantity and percentage of REM sleep noted in the recording were lower than expected

for a patient of this age. It is likely the low REM sleep quantity and percentage is secondary to the REM-sleep-suppressing effects of the amitriptyline the patient currently is taking. Tricyclic antidepressants, MAO inhibitors, and alcohol are well known to suppress REM sleep or delay its onset.

See Figure 3-8 for additional examples of REM sleep case statements.

AWAKENINGS

Definition

Not strictly defined by R&K, the term *awakenings* usually assumes that one or more epochs is scored as awake after sleep onset and before sleep offset.

General Significance

Sleep fragmentation, as defined by both arousals and awakenings from sleep, are the major consequence of many common sleep disorders seen in the sleep disorders center. Quantification of the number and duration of awakenings and arousals is an important measure of sleep quality and sleep continuity.

Alternative Term

Arousals sometimes refers to awakenings.

Possible Explanations for Atypical Number of Awakenings

A low number of awakenings may result from one or more of these factors:

- Rebound sleep (check sleep stages for high quantity and percentage).
- Hypnotic or sedative effect of medication.
- Normal sleeper.

A high number of awakenings may result from one or more of these factors:

- Sleep disorders:
  Sleep apnea.
  Periodic leg movements in sleep.
  Snoring.
- FNE.
- Drug withdrawal.
- Depression.

- Nonspecific age effects.
- Environmental disruption:
  Noise.
  Light.
  Uncomfortable mattress.
  Technician entry into sleep room.

AROUSALS

Definition

Although not defined in R&K, the American Sleep Disorders Association (ASDA) has published recommendations concerning the scoring of arousals outside the R&K standards (Table 3-2).

General Significance

Sleep fragmentation, as defined by both arousals and awakenings from sleep, is the major consequence of the most common sleep disorders seen in the sleep disorders center. R&K does not quantify brief arousals from sleep, but ASDA recommendations can be used to produce this data. Quantification of the number and duration of awakenings and arousals is an important measure of sleep quality and sleep continuity. Quantification of arousals may require additional scoring time, as it must be done separately from standard R&K scoring.

Alternative Terms

Arousals also may be called *awakenings* or *sleep fragmentation*.

Possible Explanations for Atypical Number of Arousals

A low number of arousals may result from one or more of these factors:

- Rebound sleep (check other sleep stages for high quantity and percentage).
- Hypnotic or sedative effect of medication.
- Normal sleeper.

A high number of arousals may result from one or more of these factors:

- Sleep disorders:
  Sleep apnea.
  Periodic leg movements in sleep.
  Snoring.

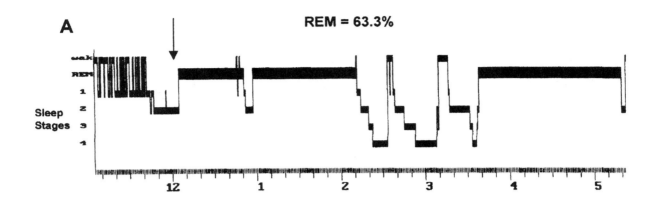

REM = 63.3%

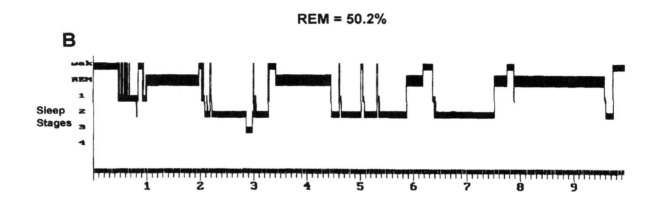

REM = 50.2%

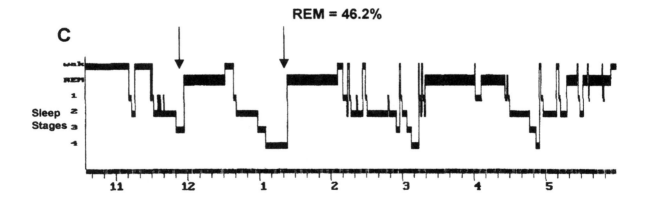

REM = 46.2%

◄ FIGURE 3-8

REM sleep case vignettes. **(A)** The sleep histogram during a nasal continuous positive airway pressure initial treatment trial. The patient was a 60-year-old white man, 5'8", 260 lbs. Prior diagnostic polysomnography revealed 805 obstructive apneas and hypopneas for an overall respiratory disturbance index of 145/hr of sleep. Low SaO_2 was 79%. Sleep during the DPSG was remarkable for 90.7% stage 1 sleep, no stage 3 or 4 (slow-wave sleep) and 6.9% (11.5 min) REM sleep. Arrow indicates start of administration of a pressure of 12.5 cm H_2O, considered to be the optimal pressure. A total of 219.5 min REM sleep was noted, for 63.3% of total sleep time. Stage 1 sleep was reduced to 8.2% total sleep time, with almost all stage 1 sleep occurring before the optimal pressure was reached. RDI at optimal pressure was 3.7/hr. Massive rebound of REM sleep does not follow predictions from experimental sleep deprivation studies. Generally, slow wave sleep rebounds first, followed by REM sleep. In the prior diagnostic sleep study, no SWS was noted, while a lower than normal percentage of REM sleep was present. The type of rebound sleep following successful NCPAP administration is unpredictable. However, sustained rebound sleep of any type should be seen as a sign that the source of prior sleep fragmentation has been reduced or eliminated. Therefore, rebound sleep, in addition to a reduced RDI, should be seen as an objective sign of successful NCPAP administration. **(B)** The sleep histogram of a DPG for a 44-year-old white woman referred for evaluation of "fatigue" and frequent awakenings from sleep. The patient previously had been diagnosed with an affective disorder by her primary care physician and prescribed 75 mg amitriptyline bid. The second dose was taken before bedtime to improve sleep quality. Over the course of two months, the patient had shown minimal improvement in her symptoms. The patient was withdrawn from the 150 mg daily dose over six days, with last dose of amitriptyline three days before date of polysomnogram. The rapid withdrawal of the medication and the failure to allow a sufficient time for REM sleep to return to normal baseline suggest that the main features of the patient's sleep are secondary to REM sleep rebound (see Figure 2-4). A total of 213 min REM sleep were noted, for 50.2% REM sleep. Latency to REM sleep was 26 min from the first 30 sec of sleep scored. Light sleep accounted for 6.6% of total sleep time and SWS sleep (stages 3 and 4) accounted for only 1.5% of total sleep time. Because the sleep noted here is almost entirely due to the effects of rebound sleep, these findings do not assist in making a diagnosis for this patient. A recommendation to repeat the study when withdrawal from amitriptyline is complete—preferably after three to four weeks—is indicated. **(C)** Sleep histogram from the DPSG for a 21-year-old white female college student who presented with complaints of AM grogginess and daytime sleepiness. DPSG was scheduled for four days after the end of final exam week. Patient described a sleep/wake schedule over the last four weeks of 3–4 hr of sleep nightly and a very irregular sleep/wake schedule for months prior to the last month. The patient reported sleeping for 6 and 8 hr on the two nights prior to the sleep study. The sleep history and the sleep histogram thus suggest a combination of both SWS and REM sleep rebound most likely due to cumulative partial sleep deprivation for at least four weeks. If sleep rebound followed the classical rebound pattern of SWS first, then this PSG represents the rebound of REM sleep after one or two nights of improved sleep. A total of 169 min REM sleep were present, along with 8.3% stage 1 sleep and 14.6% SWS. SWS is lower than expected for a patient of this age. However, the rebound sleep may be of clinical significance in that it most likely confirms that the patient has been significantly sleep deprived in the past. The fact that returning to a near normal sleep pattern of 6–8 hr sleep for the two nights prior to the DPSG did not result in normalization of sleep lends support to published findings that it is insufficient just to return to normal sleep patterns after a period of acute or partial sleep deprivation. Rather, to discharge the sleep debt fully, total sleep time must exceed the expected normal total sleep time. REM sleep latency also was shorter than expected, at 55 min. This may be secondary to either REM sleep rebound or an irregular sleep/wake schedule.

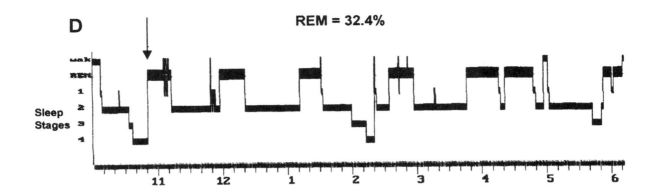

REM = 32.4%

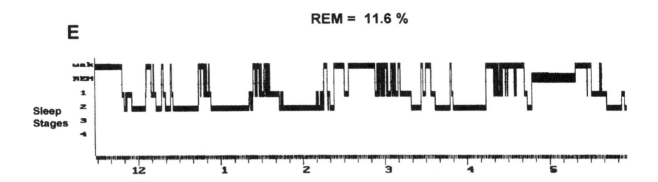

REM = 11.6 %

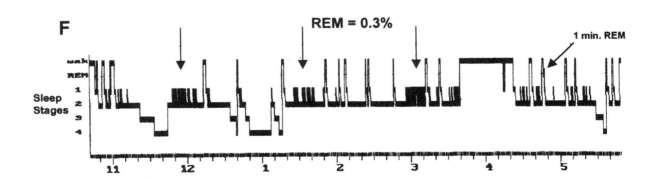

REM = 0.3%

◄ **FIGURE 3-8** *continued*

(D) The sleep histogram from an initial NCPAP treatment trial for a 71-year-old man previously diagnosed with obstructive sleep apnea. The initial DPSG showed an overall RDI of 12.5/hr of sleep, but with a REM sleep RDI of 85/hr of sleep and severely fragmented REM sleep. REM-sleep-related apneas and hypopneas were quite short, averaging 14 sec each. Only 22 min REM sleep were noted, for 7% of total sleep time. Due to the relatively short duration of REM sleep apneas and hypopneas, numerous epochs of "REM-ish" sleep were noted and scored as stage 1, during which both EEG and EMG appeared consistent with REM sleep, but eye movements did not appear before termination of the apnea or hypopnea by arousal. With administration of NCPAP, a total of 153 min REM sleep, or 32.4%, was noted with only 16 min stage 1 sleep, or 3.3% present, considerably less than expected for a man of this age. REM sleep latency was 39 min from onset of sleep and most likely is secondary to the REM sleep rebound and not secondary to depression or other medical condition. The arrow indicated the sudden and direct transition from stage 4 sleep to REM sleep with no intervening stage 2 or 3 sleep. This suggests increased "pressure" for REM sleep, consistent with the REM sleep rebound. **(E)** The sleep histogram from the DPSG of a 47-year-old man complaining of difficulty both falling asleep and maintaining sleep. Of significance, the patient recently had been diagnosed with obsessive-compulsive disorder (OCD) and initiated treatment with clomipramine 10 days earlier. This medication has a profound REM-sleep-suppressing effect (see Figures 2-4 and 2-6). REM sleep latency is delayed to 299 min, most likely secondary to the effects of this medication. REM-sleep-suppressing medications may have an effect not only on REM sleep quantity and percentage but also on REM sleep latency. Therefore, this sleep histogram does not represent a typical night of sleep. This DPSG should have been delayed for three to four weeks, until a steady-state REM percentage was reached. **(F)** The sleep histogram from the DPSG of a 45-year-old white man referred for evaluation of probable obstructive sleep apnea. An overall RDI of 65.8/hr of sleep was noted for severe sleep apnea. A single minute (two consecutive epochs) of REM sleep were noted, for a REM sleep percentage of 0.3%, well below that expected for a patient of this age. This very low REM sleep percentage may represent difficulty in scoring REM sleep due to relatively short duration of apneas and hypopneas. The first two arrows from the left indicate areas of the histogram approximately 90–180 min apart, approximating the usual REM-NREM cycle. Additionally, the sleep stages show the repeated appearance of stage 1 sleep not seen elsewhere in the histogram, again suggesting that the same process is occurring. It appeared likely that this "stage 1 sleep" actually represent early REM sleep, interrupted before all scoring criteria could be fulfilled.

TABLE 3-2
ASDA EEG Arousal Scoring Rules

An EEG arousal is

An abrupt shift in EEG frequency, which may include theta, alpha, and/or frequencies greater than 16 Hz but not spindles subject to the following rules and conditions.

EEG arousal scoring rules

1. Subjects must be asleep, defined as 10 continuous seconds or more of the indications of any stage of sleep, before an EEG arousal can be scored. Arousal scoring is independent of Rechtschaffen and Kales epoch scoring (i.e., an arousal can be scored in an epoch of recording, which would be classified as wake by Rechtschaffen and Kales criteria).
2. A minimum of 10 continuous seconds of intervening sleep is necessary to score a second arousal.
3. The EEG frequency shift must be 3 seconds or greater in duration to be scored as an arousal.
4. Arousals in NREM sleep may occur without concurrent increases in submental EMG amplitude.
5. Arousals are scored in REM sleep only when accompanied by concurrent increases in submental EMG amplitude.
6. Arousals cannot be scored based on changes in submental EMG amplitude alone.
7. Artifacts, K complexes or delta waves are not scored as arousals unless accompanied by an EEG frequency shift (as previously defined) in at least one derivation. If such activity precedes an EEG frequency shift, it is *not* included in reaching the 3-second duration criteria. When occurring within the EEG frequency shift, artifacts or delta wave activity are included in meeting duration criteria.
8. The occurrence of pen blocking artifact should be considered an arousal only if an EEG arousal pattern is contiguous. The pen blocking event can be included in reaching duration criteria.
9. Noncurrent, but contiguous, EEG and EMG changes, which were individually less than 3 seconds but together greater than 3 seconds in duration, are not scored as arousals. Intrusion of alpha activity of less than 3 seconds' duration into NREM sleep at a rate greater than one burst per 10 seconds is not scored as an EEG arousal. Three seconds of alpha sleep is not scored as an arousal unless a 10-second episode of alpha-free sleep precedes. Transitions from one stage of sleep to another are not sufficient of themselves to be scored as EEG arousals unless they meet the criteria indicated above.

Source: Modified from the Sleep Disorders Atlas Task Force. EEG arousal: Scoring rules and examples. *Sleep.* 1992;15(2):173–184.

- FNE.
- Drug withdrawal.
- Nonspecific age effects.
- Environmental disruption:
  Noise.
  Light.
  Uncomfortable mattress.
  Technician entry into sleep room.

The relatively high rates of EEG arousal noted in Table 3-3 may reflect the disrupting effects of sleeping in a laboratory rather than be features of otherwise normal sleep. Alternately, these arousals may be secondary to occult physiological events that cannot be adequately measured with current polysomnographic techniques.

Sample Statement

This recording is remarkable for the numerous, brief arousals from sleep, characterized by the appearance of high-amplitude K complexes and short runs of alpha-frequency EEG. A total 225 arousals were noted during the recording, for an arousal index of 42/hr of sleep. Approximately 50% of the arousals were secondary to the effects of snoring and irregular breathing patterns, although few apneas and hypopneas are present. The remainder of arousals has no clinical correlates in the recording, but as they appear identical in form to the other arousal patterns, they most likely also are secondary to sleep-disordered breathing. In the absence of traditionally defined apneas and hypopneas, these findings are most consistent with upper airway resistance syndrome.

SLEEP ELECTROENCEPHALOGRAM

General Significance

Certain features of the sleep EEG have a clinical significance that is not evident from standard scoring of sleep stages. While the MOE rule forces the choice of a single sleep stage for each epoch, transient features of the EEG that might be of clinical interest can be re-

TABLE 3-3
Arousals during Sleep in Asymptomatic Normal Subjects Using ASDA EEG Arousal Scoring Rules

Arousal Index (per hr sleep)	Standard Deviation or Range	Description	Reference
13.7		10 normals with a mean age of 35.8 ± 8 years with no sleep complaints	25
13.8	2.2	Normal teenagers, 10–19 yr, with no sleep complaints; RDI and PLMSI ≤5/hr of sleep on screening PSG; respiration and movement parameters not measured on experimental nights; had prior adaptation night	26
14.7	2.6	Normal young adults, 20–39 yr with no sleep complaint and RDI and PLMSI ≤5/hr of sleep on screening PSG; respiration and movement parameters not measured on experimental nights; had prior adaptation night	26
17.8	2.0	Normal middle-aged adults, 40–59 yr with no sleep complaint and RDI and PLMSI ≤5/hr of sleep on screening PSG; respiration and movement parameters not measured on experimental nights; had prior adaptation night	26
21	6–63	31 normal asymptomatic normals with a mean age of 37 yr; all screened for sleep disorders on first night in sleep laboratory without prior adaptation	27
27.1	3.3	Normal elderly, ≥60 yr, with no sleep complaint and RDI and PLMSI ≤5/hr of sleep on screening PSG; respiration and movement parameters not measured on experimental nights; had prior adaptation night	26

ported separately by the interpreter. The usual procedure of recording only one or two central lead EEG channels makes identification of focal abnormalities in the sleep EEG impossible. The interpreter should make note of atypical EEG findings, if present, without making broad statements. Sometimes, a recommendation for a full clinical EEG or return to the sleep laboratory for PSG with fuller EEG montage is appropriate.

Alpha Sleep

Alpha sleep or alpha/delta sleep is a common finding in clinical PSGs. Generally, the alpha frequency waves seen during sleep are 1–2 Hz slower than those seen during clear wakefulness. There is no specific requirement for how many alpha frequency waves must be present, but alpha waves should be clearly visible. The presence of this pattern often is associated with patient complaints of nonrestorative sleep and daytime fatigue.[28]

Sample Statement

The alpha EEG pattern is usually characteristic of drowsy wakefulness with eyes closed and disappears with the onset of sleep. However, on occasion, with the onset of sleep EEG characterized by theta and delta EEG waves, the alpha EEG pattern does not disappear but continues and becomes intermixed with the expected sleep EEG patterns. This is called an *alpha/delta* or *alpha sleep pattern*. It has been described in patients with

fibromyositis and similar disorders, psychiatric disorders, and in a variety of other unrelated disorders. It usually is associated with complaints of nonrestorative sleep and daytime fatigue. Its pathophysiology is unknown.

"Paroxysmal Delta"

Paroxysmal delta waves are a series of high-amplitude waves resembling delta EEG activity, often mixed with alpha waves and EMG artifacts. They are not followed by the suppression of EEG amplitude; frequently are seen following apneas, hypopneas, and PLMS; and are most often interpreted as arousal/artifact complexes. With treatment of the underlying cause of arousal, these bursts of delta activity almost always disappear. The uninitiated interpreter of the PSG may be tempted to describe these bursts as epileptiform or even seizure activity. If sleep apnea, PLMS, or some other repetitive process is not evident in the other channels of the PSG, a full clinical EEG should be ordered before drawing final conclusions. Out of 10,000+ PSGs, I can recall only 4 or 5 in which this type of finding eventually was determined to be epileptiform or seizure activity.

Beta

EEG in the 15–25 Hz range is not a required element of any of the standard R&K stages. Beta waves may appear in S1 and REM sleep in some individuals. More pervasive beta waves may appear due to a drug effect. On occasion, a clear drug effect may be present in the sleep EEG even though the patient denies medication use.

Epileptiform Features

The standard PSG requires only a single central derivation of EEG. It is not uncommon to see EEG features that might be consistent with sharp waves, spikes, spike and waves, and other potentially abnormal electrical activity. However, the slow recording speed and longer recording epoch (30 or 20 sec compared to 10 sec in a clinical EEG) makes identification of abnormally fast EEG activity, such as spike and sharp waves, almost impossible. Additionally, a finding of epileptiform or seizure activity almost never can be confirmed using a single EEG channel. A comment about "atypical" EEG features or a recommendation for a full clinical EEG probably is sufficient. The urge to overread the EEG should be restrained.

4

Evaluation of Cardiorespiratory Parameters

GENERAL ALGORITHM FOR INTERPRETATION SLEEP-DISORDERED BREATHING

1. Identify respiratory variables recorded.
2. Identify the method of recording.
3. Specify working definitions for different types of sleep disordered breathing.
4. Review raw polysomnogram (PSG) recording and verify that episodes of sleep-disordered breathing have been scored according to predetermined sleep laboratory procedures.
5. Examine summary data.
6. Examine histograms to permit correlation of sleep-disordered breathing with changes in sleep and other parameters.

THE MAJORITY OF THE EPOCH RULE AND SCORING RESPIRATION IN SLEEP

The majority of the epoch (MOE) rule does not apply directly to the analysis of respiratory data but has a direct effect on the computation of indexes, such as the Respiratory Disturbance Index (RDI), based on the number of episodes per hour of scored sleep. Episodes of sleep-disordered breathing may occur during epochs scored as sleep or wakefulness. Some scorers and interpreters, as well as many automated and semi-automated systems, may not include scored apneas or hypopneas in summary data if they were noted during epochs scored as wake. In the typical 30 sec scoring epoch, wake may consist of 16 sec and sleep 14 sec. As the MOE rule requires that the epoch be scored accord-

ing to the sleep stage (or wake) that occupies the majority of the epoch, significant amounts of sleep and potentially frequent episodes of sleep-disordered breathing can be eliminated from the final summary. This can lead to a dramatic reduction in the scored RDI that does not reflect the actual severity of sleep-disordered breathing in the sleep recording.

On the other hand, if numerous episodes of sleep-disordered breathing occurring during scored wakefulness are included in the final summary, the RDI (total number of apneas and hypopneas/total sleep time) can be absurdly high. Providing an RDI computed against total recording time may be more representative in this situation.

ABBREVIATIONS OF TERMINOLOGY

SDB (sleep-disordered breathing).
RDI (respiratory disturbance index).
AHI (apnea/hypopnea index).
AI (apnea index).
SaO_2 (oxygen saturation).
BPM (beats per minute, a measure of heat rate).

CLASSIFICATION OF SLEEP DISORDERED BREATHING

Definition

Episodes of sleep-disordered breathing traditionally are subdivided into categories based on their cause and form. Four general categories of sleep disordered breathing are in common use: (1) obstructive, (2) hypopnea, (3) mixed, and (4) central.

General Significance

In practice, it is essential to understand if sleep-disordered breathing is secondary to obstruction of the upper airway or due to some problem or failure of central respiratory control. For that reason, there is no practical difference between obstructive apneas and obstructive hypopneas because the upper airway pathophysiology is the same. Central apneas and central hypopneas have a distinctly different pathophysiology from obstructive events.

Methodological Concerns

Minimum Duration

Traditionally, episodes of sleep-disordered breathing must have a duration of at least 10 sec to be considered clinically meaningful events. With a respiratory rate of 12 breaths per minute, 2 breaths may occur in 10 seconds. However, this cutoff is not based on research and is essentially arbitrary. Although episodes of sleep-disordered breathing most often last longer than 10 sec in adults, there is no meaningful, scientifically based distinction from episodes of sleep-disordered breathing that last 9 or 8 sec, as is more common in children. Episodes of sleep-disordered breathing of any length, as long as they result in some perceivable consequence (e.g., arousal from sleep, transient decline in SaO_2 of 3% or more, change in heart rate, arrhythmias), should be quantified in some fashion, reported, and included in the interpretation of PSG.

Measurement Techniques

There currently is some controversy over the validity and reliability of measurement techniques.[29,30] Despite general agreement that the esophageal balloon represents the only truly quantitative measure of respiration used during sleep studies, strong opinion remains that use of semiquantitative or nonquantitative devices, such as nasal pressure or thermistors, when used with measures of respiratory effort and pulse oximetry, are more than adequate. The solution to this argument no doubt awaits future research.

Effect of Measurement Techniques on the Reliability and Validity of Respiratory Measurement

Although there is no practical or clinical difference between obstructive apneas and hypopneas, it remains common to subdivide episodes of obstructive sleep-disordered breathing as obstructive apneas or obstructive hypopneas. The interpreter who uses the obstructive hypopnea category must realize that such

definitions frequently are arbitrary, because they often depend on measurement of airflow by devices that cannot be calibrated. Very few clinical sleep laboratories use esophageal balloons. The overwhelming majority of clinical sleep laboratories use thermistors or thermocouples, devices that detect changes in air temperature at the nares and mouth. Even though these devices are often very sensitive to changes in airflow, they are not calibrated and measures of air volume cannot be derived from their signal. Therefore, airflow measured by these devices is not quantifiable. If the airflow cannot be quantitated by these devices, then insisting on a 30% or 50% reduction (a common definition of hypopneas) in an unknown volume of air has no physiological or clinical meaning. Second, thermistors and thermocouples most often are taped in position under the nose and mouth and prone to movement. Any change in position of the thermistors relative to the airways also changes the prior measurement baseline, further confusing measurement and interpretation. Finally, the use of arbitrary definitions is likely to result in a loss of meaningful clinical data. If the laboratory definition requires a 50% reduction and the sleep study shows repeated episodes of hypopnea with only a 30% reduction, it is very likely that the sleep study will underestimate the actual clinical severity. The thoughtful sleep-disorders clinician should consider a more pragmatic approach. Consider the following definition taken from one of the most influential research papers on sleep apnea:

> An abnormal breathing event during objectively measured sleep was defined according to the commonly used clinical criterion of either a complete cessation of airflow lasting 10 seconds or more (apnea) or a discernible reduction in respiratory airflow accompanied by a decrease of 4% or more in oxyhemoglobin saturation (hypopnea).[31(p. 1232)]

The clear implication is that, since data acquisition techniques are imperfect, the sleep-disorders clinician should look for all meaningful data regardless of the definition.

This problem can have a direct effect on the measurement, reporting, and interpretation of central sleep apneas and hypopneas. Central sleep apnea is defined by the absence of airflow and respiratory interruption in control of breathing due to changes in neural respiratory centers or blood gases. Respiratory effort is reduced or ceases, and airflow is reduced or ceases proportionally. Central sleep-disordered breathing implies that the upper airway is patent and not involved in the reduction in airflow. Insufficiently sensitive sensors may not show that continuing respiratory effort is present, resulting in inappropriate diagnosis and treatment.

RESPIRATORY DISTURBANCE INDEX

Definition

Generally includes all scored apneas and hypopneas divided by total sleep time in hours (apneas and hypopneas/hr of sleep). However, the RDI may be defined to include other types of sleep-disordered breathing, including snores or snore resulting in arousals.

Alternate Terminology

The RDI sometimes is called the *apnea/hypopnea index* (AHI).

General Significance

The RDI is a general metric for the overall frequency of episodes of sleep-disordered breathing and often is used to specify the level of severity.

Methodological Concerns

Computation
The RDI can be affected by the MOE rule, resulting in either an inappropriate reduction in RDI, if apneas and hypopneas occurring during scored wakefulness are excluded or an inappropriate increase in RDI, if apneas and hypopneas are included in the computation but no adjustments are made.

Relationship to Severity
The RDI often is the primary measurement used to determine the severity of sleep apnea in a recording. RDI most often is arbitrarily divided into the following four categories of severity:

Normal: <5/hr
Mild: 5–19/hr
Moderate: 20–40/hr
Severe: >40/hr

These categories are not the result of data-based research and are not related to outcome measures. The use of generic terms such as *mild* also may be misconstrued as meaning clinically insignificant. As noted in Table 4-1, even mild obstructive sleep apnea can result in significant and measurable changes in cognitive and psychosocial functioning. The PSG interpreter should look not only to the RDI but the degree of sleep fragmentation, severity of hypoxemia, and presence of cardiac arrhythmias before making any final determination of severity.

OXYGEN SATURATION

Definition

Oxygen saturation (SaO_2) refers to the quantity of oxygen carried by hemoglobin in the blood. When measured by a pulse oximeter, it sometimes is referred to as SpO_2. Oxygen in the blood is bound primarily to hemoglobin although very small quantities may be dissolved in other blood cells as well.

Pulse oximeters typically emit light of 2 wavelengths through the arterial bed of the finger, earlobe, or other location. A detector on the other side of the finger, earlobe, or other location measures the attenuated light. Early nonpulse oximeters were unable to distinguish light absorbed by tissues and hemoglobin not in arterial blood. The early devices compensated for this problem by heating tissues and using numerous wavelengths. Modern pulse oximeters were devised when it was noted that the amount of light absorbed by hemoglobin varied with each pulse. The absorption values noted during the base and peak of each pulse therefore can be attributed to arterial blood alone. Modern pulse oximeters measure functional saturation (oxyhemoglobin/ (oxyhemoglobin + reduced or deoxyhemoglobin) × 100%). Other species of hemoglobin are not directly measured but are assumed to be present in very low percentages (<2%). When other species of hemoglobin are present in higher percentages, they may cause measurement errors.

The normal range of oxygen saturation is 90–100%, with values below this level labeled as *hypoxemia*.

General Significance

SaO_2 often is the only calibrated, quantifiable measure of respiration during the polysomnogram. SaO_2 as measured by pulse oximeter provides information regarding amount of oxygen bound to hemoglobin only and not (1) the oxygen content in blood, (2) quantity of oxygen dissolved in blood, (3) respiratory rate or tidal volume, or (4) cardiac output of blood pressure.[49]

Methodological Concerns

SaO_2 may vary significantly, depending on the individual pulse oximeter, laboratory setting, and patient. Interpreters should consult their oximeter manual or

TABLE 4-1
Respiratory Disturbance Index: Associated Findings

Mean RDI	Standard Deviation or Range	Associated Findings and Consequences	Reference
>5	5–15	Compared to men without sleep-disordered breathing, 4.2 times more likely to have a car accident in 5 yr	32
5		Increased risk for hypertension, odds ratio 1.21 (CI 1.09–1.34)	33
7.5	5–9.9	After 4 weeks of NCPAP treatment, statistically significant increase in driving simulation scores, mood, and SF-36 score, total symptom scores	34
8.7	5.5	Statistically significant impairment of quality of life or psychosocial functioning compared to matched normal controls (48.1 ± 17 yrs) with an RDI of 3.7 ± 3.4/hr	35
10.0	3	After 4 weeks of NCPAP treatment, statistically significant increase in subjective sleepiness, performance, mood, and SF-36 scores	34
10.3	12.2	After 6 months of CPAP treatment, increase in mean Multiple Sleep Latency Test (MSLT) from 4.9 ± 2.3 to 8.9 ± 4.0 min, however, measures of planning ability and manual dexterity remain abnormal—chronic deficits resulting from severe hypoxia	36
11.1		After 4 weeks of NCPAP treatment, increased symptom score, mental flexibility, and mood	34
15		Significant impairment of psychomotor efficiency equal to 5 yr additional age or 50% of the expected decrease from sedating medication use	37
15		Increased risk for hypertension, odds ratio 1.75 (CI 1.28-2.40)	33
>15		Compared to adults without sleep-disordered breathing, 7.3 times more likely to have a multiple car accident in 5 yr	32
17.0	4.9	Statistically significant deficits compared to normal controls in visual vigilance and working memory but not MSLT or subjective alertness	38
21.2	7.2	Significant decreases in mean MSLT and various cognitive measures	39
28	7–120	Significantly increased driving simulator performance after 4 weeks CPAP treatment	40
30		Increased risk for hypertension, odds ratio 3.01 (CI 1.65–1.74)	33
38	27	General health status statistically worse than matched normal controls (45 ± 13 yr)	41
40		Increase in car accidents and disability compared to normal controls	42
41	4.5	Statistically significant deficits in executive functions, such as attention, short-term memory, learning ability, planning, verbal fluency; hypothesized to be secondary to frontal lobe deficits suggestive of hypoxic damage	43
46.7	32.4	Treatment with NCPAP for two nights (RDI of 8.2 ± 11.8/hr) resulted in increased measures of alertness but not all cognitive deficits were immediately reversible—effects of hypoxia	44
57	38	Seven times more likely to have car accidents	45
65.6	25.5	Statistically decreased cerebral vascular reactivity to hypercapnia compared to normal controls (mean age 54 yr)	46
68.8	12.9	Significant decreases in MSLT and various cognitive functions compared to normal controls; additional decreases in general intelligence measures, executive functions, and psychomotor performance compared to moderate OSA (RDI = 21.2/hr), attributed to more significant hypoxia	39
83	20	Mean age 46 ± 11 yr; decreased driving simulator performance compared to control normals	47
86	14	Impaired attention, concentration, problem solving, memory compared to a group with RDI of 43/hr; degree of hypoxia reported to be most statistically significant factor	48

Note: This table provides a listing of selected research and clinical studies with associated psychological and medical findings. Although these findings are listed by RDI, the associated finding may be secondary to hypoxia or other cardiopulmonary consequences of sleep apnea.

manufacturer for specific information about the pulse oximeter in use in their sleep laboratory.

Potential problems include:[50,51]

- Poor perfusion:
  Cold temperature.
  Hypotension.
  Hypovolemia.
  Cardiogenic shock.
- Inadequate light transmission:
  Tissue edema.
  Skin color.
  Tissue thickness.
  Improper placement of probe.
- Small pulse amplitude.
- Inadequate pulse due to cardiac arrhythmias.
- Motion.
  Gross movements, loss of signal.
  Vibrations in range of heart rate (0.5–3.5 Hz), inaccurate signals.
- Excessive light:
  Xenon and infrared lights, high likelihood of interference.
  Intense daylight.
  Fluorescent lights.
  Incandescent lights.
- Venous pulsation. (Pulse oximeters interpret all pulsations as arterial in origin.)
- Dyshemoglobins. Most pulse oximeters use only 2 wavelengths of light and are intended to detect oxyhemoglobin and reduced hemoglobin or deoxyhemoglobin. Other species of hemoglobin that absorb light at similar wavelengths—carboxyhemoglobin and methemoglobin—may interfere with accurate measurement. Carboxyhemoglobins resulting from CO_2 poisoning, smoke inhalation, or heavy smoking can account for >10% hemoglobin and result in significantly increased SaO_2 values.
- Vital dyes, nail polish, and pigmentation.
- Response delay:
  Finger probe, 10–30 sec.
  Earlobe, 5–10 sec.
- Accuracy. Most modern pulse oximeters have an accuracy of ±2% between values of 70–99% and ±3% from 50–69%, as calibrated with human volunteers. However, measured SaO_2 has been reported to become increasingly inaccurate below 85%, and 80% may be the lowest accurate value.
- Medical conditions:
  CO poisoning.
  Smoke inhalation.
  Heavy smoking.

- Sampling rate. SaO_2 values most often are averaged over periods from 3 to 10 sec. Longer averaging periods may be useful in reducing motion artifact but inappropriate for sleep studies (Figure 4-1).

Transient versus Chronic Declines in SaO_2

All-night measurement of SaO_2 during polysomnograms typically produces one of the following four patterns of SaO_2 (Figure 4-2):

1. Normal SaO_2. SaO_2 ≥90% with no state or body position shift but may include brief motion-related artifact.
2. Short-term drop in SaO_2 <90%. Drops in SaO_2 usually last minutes or the duration of rapid eye movement (REM) sleep, due to supine body position or artifacts resulting from problems with equipment or patient compliance. SaO_2 returns to ≥90% when these factors are not present.
3. Chronic or long-term hypoxemia (SaO_2 ≤90%). This condition is present either only during sleep or during all 24 hours and most often is related to chronic lung disease or other serious medical disorders.
4. Repetitive O_2 desaturation. Drops in SaO_2 of ≥2–4% (depending on specific sleep laboratory's definition and equipment) usually last <60 sec. SaO_2 returns to ≥90% thereafter. This most often is related to the effects of upper airway obstruction.

Effects of Hypoxemia on Physiology and Cognitive Functioning

Hypoxemia is well known to affect both physiological and cognitive functioning. Numerous studies have been performed, especially on the effects of altitude and consequent hypoxia on cognitive function. However, very few studies have been performed on the effects of repetitive declines and rises in SaO_2 compared to the chronic low SaO_2 seen in altitude studies. No experimental studies of the effects of rapidly increasing and decreasing SaO_2 in human subjects currently is available. The general effects of chronic hypoxia on the brain can be seen in Table 4-2, the data for which was taken from the classic Gibson et al. study of mild hypoxia. Its applicability to the repetitive periods of hypoxia of sleep apnea is unknown.

Hypoxemia and Rapid Eye Movement Sleep

As noted in the RDI section, sleep-disordered breathing and associated hypoxemia often are exacerbated

A

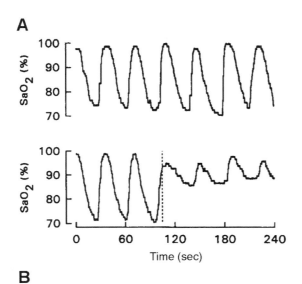

B

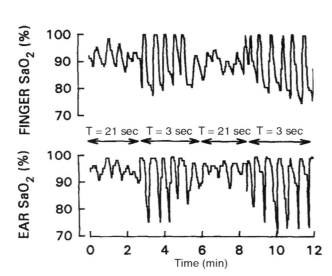

FIGURE 4-1

Effects of averaging time and sensor location of SaO_2. **(A)** Modern pulse oximeters generally come with several settings for averaging time. A long averaging time might be useful in cases where there is significant movement, such as in a test involving exertion or exercise. However, during sleep studies, the averaging time should be relative short to acquire data from rapid apnea/hypopnea-related O_2 desaturations. **(B)** The effects of averaging time and placement of the oximetry probe on the finger or ear: $t = 21$ is a long time response or averaging that is not appropriate for sleep recording, and $t = 3$ is a short response time or averaging time that is appropriate for sleep recording. (Reprinted with permission from Farre R, Montserrat JM, Ballester E, Hernandez L, Rotger M, Navajas D. Importance of the pulse oximeter averaging time when measuring oxygen desaturation in sleep apnea. *Sleep.* 1998;21(4):386–390.)

TABLE 4-2

Effect of Hypoxia on Functioning of the Human Brain

SaO_2 (%)	Altitude (ft)	Equivalent FiO_2 (%)	PaO_2 (mm Hg)	$PaCO_2$ (mm Hg)	Clinical Status
97	Sea level	21	95	38	Normal
91-81	10–15,000	14-11	60-45	36-34	Impaired concentration, impaired short-term memory, hyperventilation
81-67	15,000–20,000	11-9	45-35	34-30	Lethagy, euphoria, irritability, hallucinations, impaired critical judgment, muscular incoordination
67	>20,000	9	35	30	Loss of consciousness

Source: Modified from Gibson GE, Pulsinelli W, Blass J, Duffy TE. Brain dysfunction in mild to moderate hypoxia. *Am J Med.* 1981;70:1247–1254.

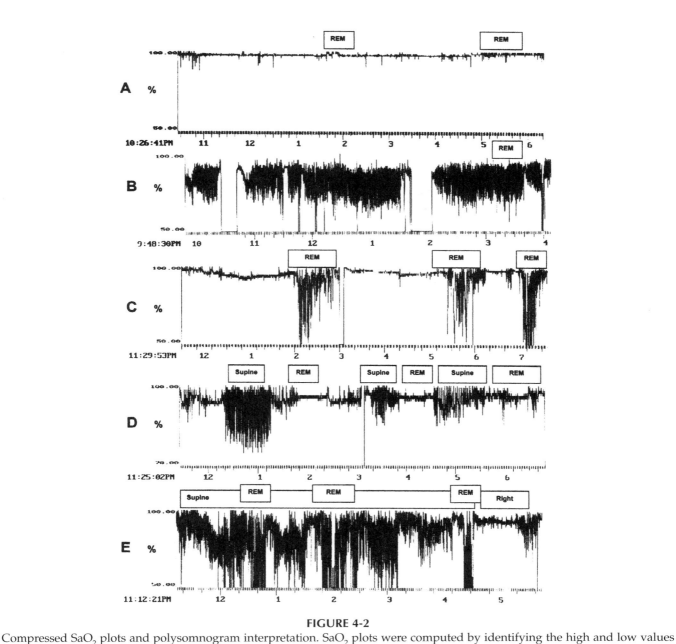

FIGURE 4-2

Compressed SaO$_2$ plots and polysomnogram interpretation. SaO$_2$ plots were computed by identifying the high and low values during each 30 sec epoch. When SaO$_2$ is presented in this way there often is a distinct pattern that can assist in the interpretation of data. **(A)** Normal SaO$_2$. Compressed all-night plot of SaO$_2$ for a 28-year-old patient under evaluation for excessive daytime sleepiness due to probable insufficient sleep. Changes in plot show only 1–3% reductions in SaO$_2$ with no significant changes during REM sleep. Changes at the left of the plot occurred with movement. **(B)** Severe, repetitive O$_2$ desaturations. Compressed plot of SaO$_2$ associated with severe obstructive sleep apnea a 45-year-old man. RDI = 97/hr of sleep. No changes apparent during REM sleep. Blank areas occurred with patient out of bed. **(C)** Severe, REM-sleep-related O$_2$ desaturations. A 62-year-old woman with an overall RDI of 20.2/hr of sleep but with a REM RDI of 57.0/hr of sleep. As REM sleep cannot be manipulated voluntarily by the patient or members of the technical staff, the theoretical maximum for REM-sleep-related episodes of sleep-disordered breathing should be equal to the REM RDI multiplied by the maximum expected REM quantity (in hours) for a patient of this age. **(D)** Severe, intermittent, positional O$_2$ desaturations. Episodes of sleep-disordered breathing and associated O$_2$ desaturation in a 39-year-old man occurring almost exclusively in the supine position and not in REM sleep. The overall RDI was 47.2/hr. The REM sleep RDI was 8.0/hr and the supine RDI was 62.4/hr. As body position can be manipulated by patients or members of the technical staff, the maximum number of episodes of sleep-disordered breathing is limited only by the number of hours the patient sleeps in the supine position. Additionally, the failure of REM sleep to cause any significant exacerbation of sleep-disordered breathing is unusual and suggests that REM sleep may not always be an exacerbating factor. Different patients may have different exacerbating conditions. **(E)** Severe, positional O$_2$ desaturations with REM sleep exacerbation. All-night plot of SaO$_2$ in a 42-year-old man who spent the majority of the recording in the supine position. REM sleep resulted in further exacerbation, with SaO$_2$ declining to 32%. Values below 50% are plotted due to the likelihood they are inaccurate. When the patient moved to the right lateral decubitus position late in the recording, the RDI declined from 85/hr of sleep to 12/hr of sleep.

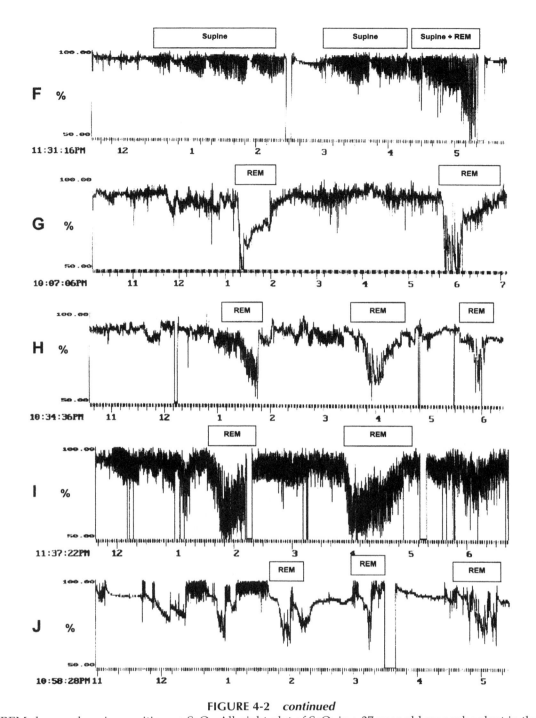

FIGURE 4-2 *continued*

(F) Effect of REM sleep and supine position on SaO_2. All-night plot of SaO_2 in a 37-year-old man who slept in the supine position for 80% of the recording. REM sleep appeared for the first time at 4:30 AM with resulting significant increase in hypoxemia to <50%. **(G)** REM sleep hypoxemia in a 65-year-old man with recently diagnosed chronic obstructive pulmonary disease (COPD) and mild sleep apnea. Note, during the first REM period, just after 1 AM, the sudden decline in SaO_2, from low 90s to <50% in less than 5 min. The second period of REM sleep, starting just before 6 AM, shows several transient increases in SaO_2 into the 70s. **(H)** REM sleep hypoxemia with moderate obstructive sleep apnea (OSA). A 57-year-old woman with no history of lung or heart disease. During REM sleep, O_2 desaturation and repetitive apneas and hypopneas were noted. However, brief terminating arousals from apneas and hypopneas resulted in <5% increase in SaO_2 and, on return to sleep, SaO_2 continued to decline rapidly. **(I)** REM sleep hypoxemia with severe OSA and no history of lung or heart disease. Similar to case H, with an RDI of 110/hr sleep and significant O_2 desaturation in both REM and NREM sleep. **(J)** Severe hypoxemia with moderate OSA. Compressed plot of SaO_2 in a 5'6", 380-lb man with COPD during administration of bilevel positive airway pressure (BiPAP) at 17.5 cm H_2O IPAP (inspiratory positive airway pressure) and 7.5 cm H_2O EPAP (expiratory positive airway pressure) with 8 l/min supplemental O_2 administered via the nasal mask. Despite this treatment, significant declines in SaO_2 were present. Patient admitted to inpatient medical service of hospital the next day.

by the presence of REM sleep. In cases where sleep is severely fragmented by sleep-disordered breathing, hypoxemia may be useful as a check on REM sleep stage scoring.

A close review of the sections of the PSGs in Figures 4-3 and 4-4 marked areas 1 and 2 show that, although rapid eye movements were few, many epochs in these areas indeed could be scored as REM sleep. REM sleep thus increased from 50.5 min and 13.9% of total sleep time (TST) to 110 min and 28.9% of TST.

SNORING

General Significance

Snoring is an easy-to-measure marker of sleep-disordered breathing and upper airway resistance.

Methodological Concerns

Measurement of snoring usually is not the result of a calibrated measurement in the standard polysomnogram. Snoring rarely is calibrated against a known decibel scale and, as a result, is not easily quantifiable. Presleep patient calibrations, during which the patient is asked to simulate a snore, often provide the only benchmark of whether a snore actually produces a change in the polysomnographic tracing. In the absence of a calibration against a known sound, the snoring measurement may not help differentiate between soft and loud snoring.

Snoring may be worsened by

- Sleep deprivation, total or partial cumulative.
- Alcohol.
- CNS depressant medication.
- Airway edema.
- Nasal congestion.
- Supine body position.
- Sleeping without head elevated.
- Nasal septal deviation or other abnormalities of the nose or upper airway.

or improved by

- Nasal continuous positive airway pressure (NCPAP).
- Nasal decongestants.
- Nasal dilators, external or internal.
- Oral appliances.
- Body position other than supine.
- Elevation of head.
- Absence of prior sleep deprivation.

Existing Definition of Snoring Severity

International Classification of Sleep Disorders
The following is modified from *International Classification of Sleep Disorders,* Diagnostic Classification Steering Committee, M. J. Thorpy, Chairman:[52]

Mild: Snoring occurs less than nightly, and only in the supine body position.
Moderate: Snoring occurs nightly and occasionally disturbs others. Usually abolished by change in body position.
Severe: Snoring occurs nightly, disturbs others, and is not altered by change in body position. Bed partners may have to sleep in another room due to the loudness of the snoring.

This definition does not depend on objective measurement of sound. In practice, the severity of snoring often is determined by the night shift polysomnographic technologist. The interpreter should have an understanding of the sleep technologist's subjective scale for rating snoring severity.

PARADOXICAL BREATHING

Definition

Paradoxical breathing (PB) is an out of phase movement of the chest wall and abdomen.

General Significance

When not secondary to a medical condition, paradoxical breathing can be seen as an alternative measure of upper airway resistance or obstruction in the absence of traditionally defined apneas or hypopneas.

Methodological Concerns

Detection of paradoxical breathing during sleep requires simultaneous measurement of both abdominal and chest wall movement. A calibration during clear wakefulness should show the absence of paradoxical breathing.

Conditions Characterized by Paradoxical Breathing

- Obstructive sleep apnea.
- Upper airway resistance syndrome.
- Pulmonary disorders.

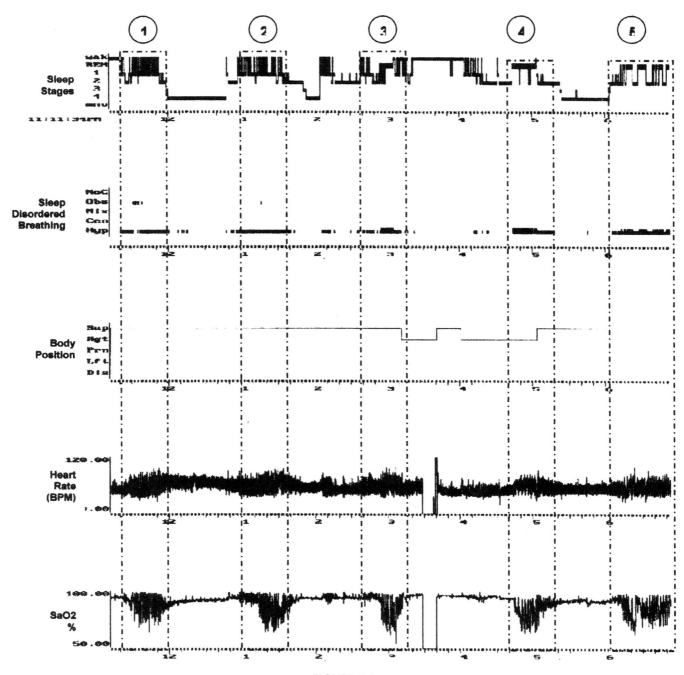

FIGURE 4-3

Effects of REM and NREM sleep of OSA and hypoxia. Histograms from the PSG of a 42-year-old woman with severe obstructive sleep apnea. The overall RDI was 64.6/hr of sleep, but sleep-disordered breathing was much more severe during REM sleep for a REM RDI of 120/hr of sleep. An additional remarkable finding is that significant deep sleep also is present, with 105 min stage 3 and 4 sleep. During stage 3 and 4 sleep, apneas and hypopneas were absent although snoring continued. As seen in the bottom SaO_2 plot, REM sleep was associated with significant hypoxia, see areas 3, 4, and 5. These appear to be periods of typical REM-sleep-related hypoxia. However, the periods of O_2 desaturation found in hatch marked areas #1 and 2 appear identical to those in 3, 4, and 5, but are not associated with scored REM sleep. The timing of these periods of O_2 desaturation, starting with area 1, appears to be about every 90–120 min, suggesting the REM-NREM period. This strongly suggests that, although REM sleep was not scored during areas 1 and 2, these indeed are periods of REM sleep. The technical staff was advised to review this highly fragmented sleep to determine if scorable REM sleep was present.

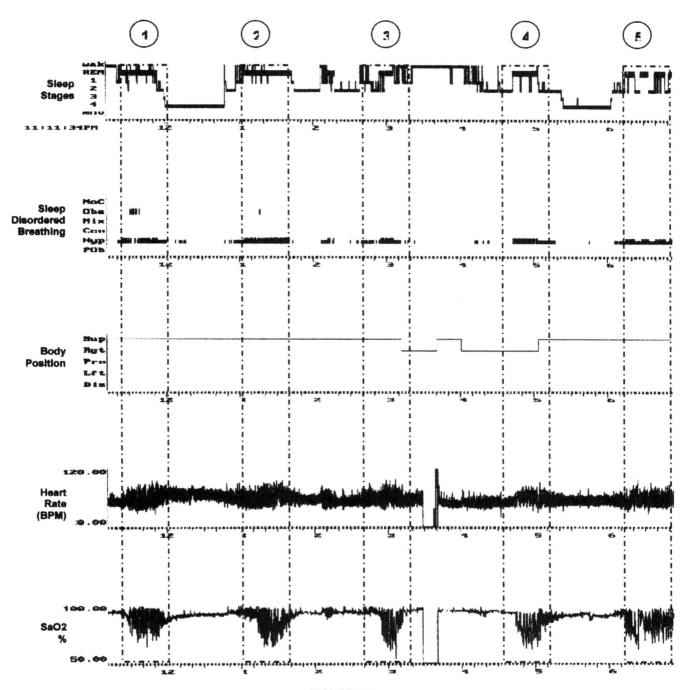

FIGURE 4-4
Episodic hypoxia as a marker of REM sleep.

CARDIAC ARRHYTHMIAS

General Significance

Cardiac arrhythmias are common findings both during normal sleep and in association with sleep disorders such as sleep apnea. Cardiac arrhythmias noted during PSGs may be

- Non-sleep dependent appearing with no specific relationship to sleep or wakefulness.
- Sleep dependent, appearing only during sleep.
- REM sleep dependent, appearing when vagal tone is high.
- Phasic REM sleep dependent, appearing only during bursts of rapid eye movements.
- Hypoxia dependent, appearing during periods of hypoxia.
- REM sleep and hypoxia dependent, appearing during periods of REM-sleep-associated hypoxia, particularly in association with obstructive sleep apnea.

Methodological Concerns

- The majority of polysomnographic recordings do not make use of full ECG montages. Rather, a single lead, most often a lead I or modified lead I, is used with the understanding that subtle changes in the ECG cannot be detected.
- No generally accepted classification of cardiac arrhythmias is available to guide clinical decision making for sleep medicine specialists.[53] The International Classification of Sleep Disorders[52] provides diagnostic and severity criteria for only one type of cardiac arrhythmia, the REM sleep-related sinus arrest, perhaps because it is considered a separate diagnostic entity. A review of the diagnostic and severity criteria for REM sleep-related sinus arrest provides a starting point for thinking about the interpretation of cardiac arrhythmias in general during the PSG. The diagnostic criteria for REM sleep-related sinus arrest is that polysomnographic monitoring demonstrates asystole lasting greater than 2.5 sec, occurring solely in REM sleep. The severity of REM sleep-related sinus arrest is classified as:[52]

Mild: Episodes of sinus arrest of to 3 sec duration, typically occurring more than twice per night.
Moderate: Episodes of sinus arrest of 3–5 sec duration, occurring several times per night.
Severe: Episodes of sinus arrest of greater than 5 sec duration, occurring five or more times per night.

- Of course, this deals only with one type of cardiac arrhythmia and may not be applicable to other types of cardiac arrhythmias seen during sleep.

In the absence of a generally accepted classification for all cardiac arrhythmias, one—not entirely satisfactory—alternative is to look at the recently published guidelines of the American College of Cardiology (ACC) and American Heart Association (AHA)[54] regarding the implantation of cardiac pacemakers and antiarrhythmia devices. If these cardiac arrhythmias are thought to be of sufficient danger to require the placement of a pacemaker or implantable cardioverter-defibrillator (ICD), then they are likely to be of concern to the sleep medicine specialist. The use of these guidelines is limited by the assumption that much more clinical and testing data are available to the cardiologist than the usual single-lead ECG found in sleep recordings. Additionally, these guidelines assume that the cardiac arrhythmias have occurred in wakefulness. As noted previously, cardiac arrhythmias may be state specific.

Nevertheless, these guidelines represent a source of general information of which cardiac arrhythmias are considered severe enough to require invasive treatment if they occur during wakefulness. They are included as general guidelines only. When in doubt as to the significance of cardiac arrhythmias occurring during sleep, seek a cardiologic consultation.

The following are cardiac arrhythmias for which pacemaker or ICD implantation were found to be useful, effective, or beneficial. The cardiac arrhythmias listed are limited to those that might be identified using the single-lead ECG common to most diagnostic PSGs.

1. Third-degree AV block associated with
   Asystole >3.0 sec in an awake, asymptomatic patient.
   Escape rate <40 beats per minute.
2. Third-degree AV block with chronic bifascicular and trifascicular block.
3. Second-degree AV Mobitz Type II with chronic bifascicular and trifascicular block.
4. Congenital third-degree AV block with wide QRS escape rhythm.
5. Second-degree AV Mobitz Type II block in patients without bifascicular and trifascicular block.

The guidelines also suggest that the following cardiac arrhythmias should be considered within the normal range:

1. Bradycardia with rates >30 beats/min.
2. Sinus pause <3 sec.
3. AV nodal Wenckebach block.

A recent review of bradyarrhythmias by Mangrum and DiMarco stated that the following arrhythmias occur frequently enough in sleep to be considered within normal limits:[55]

1. Heart rates of 30–35 beats/min.
2. Sinoatrial block of ≤2.5 sec.
3. Junctional rhythms.
4. First- and second-degree AV nodal block.
5. Pauses ≤4 sec during atrial fibrillation.

The authors further note that, "When bradycardia, even if extreme, is present only during sleep, pacing is usually not indicated."[55]

A second, more common concern regarding brady-arrhythmias during sleep is whether the cause of the arrhythmias is reversible. This generally refers to cardiac arrhythmias that occur only secondary to obstructive apneas and hypoxia, especially during REM sleep. Generally, *reversible* refers to the fact that these cardiac arrhythmias usually are eliminated with successful treatment of the obstructive sleep apnea; hence, the potential for relatively easy treatment. Unfortunately, this does not address the question of the potential danger of these cardiac arrhythmias to the patient before the sleep apnea is successfully treated or to the patient who is noncompliant with treatment. This is an especially important question in light of the relatively poor level of treatment compliance reported for patients treated with nasal continuous positive airway pressure (CPAP) for sleep apnea.

Ventricular arrhythmias also may occur during sleep. However, even less information is available regarding their potential severity or danger during sleep. A possible source of information regarding interpretation of severity of ventricular arrhythmias comes from the classic paper by Lown and Wolf [56] describing the relationship between ventricular prema-ture beats (VPBs) and sudden cardiac death in patients with coronary heart disease. Lown and Wolf created a grading system for ventricular arrhythmias that has been modified by others. Table 4-3 is one variant of this system that combines not only the frequency of ventricular arrhythmias but their form as well. Again, this table is presented only as a general guideline to severity and is not specific to sleep.

The presence of cardiac arrhythmia during sleep always should be considered before making severity statements for obstructive sleep apnea. The presence of cardiac arrhythmias thought to be potentially dangerous should be commented on and may result in an increase in severity levels.

BODY POSITION

Definition

The body position is assumed by the patient during the PSG. Generally, the description is limited to a supine, prone, right lateral decubitus, or left lateral decubitus position, although some body position detection devices measure eight or more positions.

General Significance

The body position noted may significantly affect the frequency, duration, and severity of sleep-disordered breathing.

Methodological Concerns

Measurement in the Sleep Laboratory

The sleep laboratory measurement of body position can be performed using a variety of sensors. These sensors generally are attached to a belt or directly to the patient. They vary in size and number of positions

TABLE 4-3

Classification of Ventricular Arrhythmias by Frequency and Form

Frequencies	Forms
Class 0—Nil	Class A—Uniform morphology, unifocal
Class 1—Rare (<1/hr)	Class B—Multiform, multifocal
Class 2—Infrequent (1–9/hr)	Class C—Repetitive forms, couplets, salvos, repetitive responses (3–5 consecutive ventricular complexes)
Class 3—Intermediate (10–29/hr)	Class D—Nonsustained ventricular tachycardia (>6 consecutive ventricular complexes to runs <30 sec)
Class 4—Frequent (>30/hr)	Class E—Sustained ventricular tachycardia (runs of ventricular complexes >30 sec)

Source: Reprinted with permission from Myerburg RJ, Kessler KM, Luceri RM, Zaman L, Trohman RG, Estes D, Castellanos A. Classification of ventricular arrhythmias based on parallel hierarchies of frequency and form. *Am J Cardiology.* 1984;54:1355–1358.

that can be measured. Body position alternatively can be observed directly by the polysomnographic technologist via closed-circuit infrared TV. Body position sensors have the advantage of not requiring the PSG technologist's attention. On the other hand, even body position sensors that can record eight body positions may not be able to accurately describe a patient lying in a twisted position or with an unusual head position.

Sleep in the Laboratory versus at Home

It is common sleep laboratory wisdom, often supported by the patient's comments the morning after sleep studies, that patients could not sleep in their usual body positions due to the electrodes, sensors, or NCPAP mask. Generally, they report spending more time in a supine position in the sleep laboratory than at home. The limited number of studies in this area support this contention. A study of patients with mild-to-moderate sleep apnea in the sleep laboratory both with and without electrodes and sensors attached found a 56% increase in sleep in the supine position on the nights when patients slept with electrodes and sensors. In a study in which patients with sleep apnea were studied both at home and in the sleep laboratory, sleep in the supine position was reported to be much lower at home (10.4%) than in the sleep laboratory (60.8%).[57]

Effect of Body Position on Sleep Apnea

Body position, and especially the time spent supine, are potentially critical because of the effects on sleep apnea. Sleep apnea that occurs primarily in the supine position often is referred to as *positional sleep apnea*. Obstructive sleep apnea may occur only with the patient in the supine position and may be exacerbated by a change to the supine position.

Diagnostic Problems with Body Position

Body position introduces a variable that is difficult to control for. The laboratory technical staff can request that the patient assume certain body positions during the sleep study for certain periods of time. However, it generally is unknown how this relates to the patient's usual habits at home. Nevertheless, especially during NCPAP titrations or split night protocols, it may be necessary to have the patient sleep in the supine position for at least a short period of time, so that its effect on sleep apnea and subsequently on the NCPAP pressure level required for treatment can be noted. Of course, requests that the patient sleep in the supine position may not be sufficient to generate the most severe sleep apnea. It generally is acknowledged that sleep apnea is likely to be most severe when the patient is sleeping in the supine position during REM sleep (see Figures 4-5 and 4-6 and Table 4-4). While the technician can request the patient to change into a supine position, REM sleep cannot be conjured up whenever the technician desires it. Of course, the technician may request the patient to remain in the supine position until REM sleep appears.

The breakdown in Table 4-4 shows that the most severe apnea occurs with the patient supine and in REM sleep. However, the highest RDI is not present during REM sleep because REM-sleep-related apneas and hypopneas have longer durations and so a lower RDI (with longer durations fewer events can occur per hour). If the patient had not slept in the supine position and little or no REM sleep had occurred, the interpreter might have had no option other than to say this recording is consistent with mild obstructive sleep apnea. This should be followed by some type of modifying statement to the effect that, if REM sleep or a supine position had been noted, more severe sleep apnea might have been diagnosed.

When body position has a clear effect on the frequency of episodes of sleep-disordered breathing, the interpreter has a difficult decision. Often this has to do with reporting the laboratory study in one way, while warning that it may not be typical of sleep and breathing in the home.

DETERMINATION OF SEVERITY RATING OF SLEEP DISORDERED BREATHING

General Considerations

It is important to remember that the severity rating that is part of the interpretation of PSGs may not necessarily be the severity rating of the final diagnosis of the patient. The final diagnosis may—and should—take into account other factors, daytime sleepiness often being the most important. The use of specific

TABLE 4-4

Statistics for REM and Supine Position Effects in Figure 4-6

	Body Position	
	Supine	Right
REM sleep		
Respiratory disturbance index	75	45
Low SaO$_2$	<50%	85%
NREM sleep		
Respiratory disturbance index	85	15
Low SaO$_2$	82%	92%

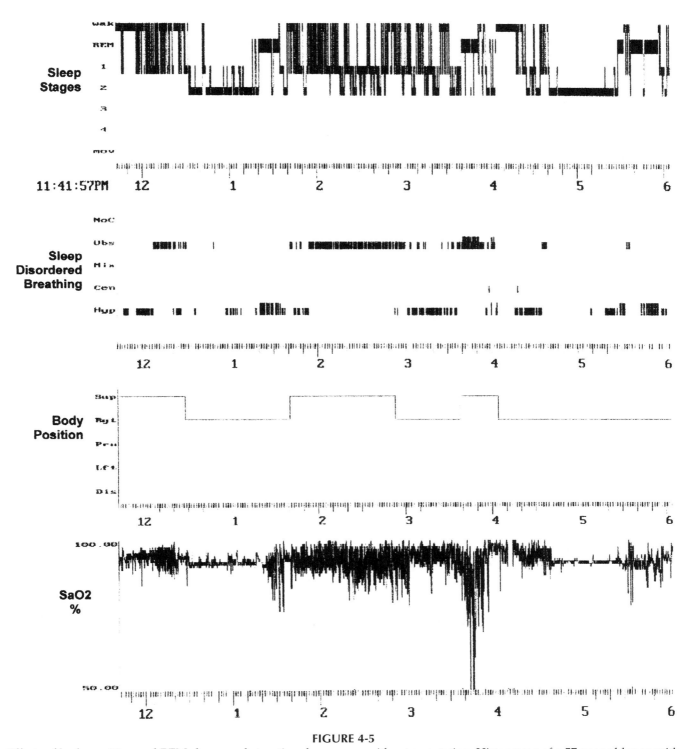

FIGURE 4-5

Effects of body position and REM sleep on obstructive sleep apnea without annotation. Histograms of a 57-year-old man with severe obstructive sleep apnea. The overall RDI was 81.9/hr of sleep with O_2 desaturation to <50%.

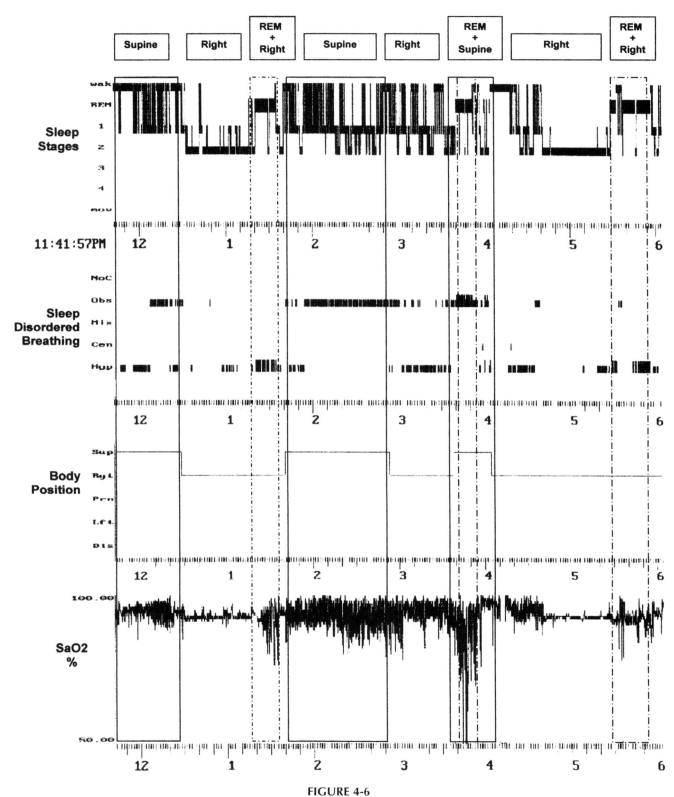

FIGURE 4-6

Effects of body position and REM sleep on obstructive sleep apnea annotated. These are the same histograms as in Figure 4-5 analyzed by body position and presence of REM or NREM sleep. Table 4-4 provides the numbers data to go with the figure.

numerical cutoffs should be used with caution. The following caution appears in the initial sections of the *International Classification of Sleep Disorders*. Clearly this caution is applicable to the interpretation of all PSG data and not just to cardiopulmonary data used to diagnose obstructive sleep apnea:

> In a few disorders, additional information is supplied to aid in determining severity, such as the number of movements per hour of sleep (PLM index) in periodic limb movement disorder. These criteria should be considered in addition to the criteria for the primary symptom of either insomnia or excessive sleepiness. However, for the majority of the disorders, the classification committee purposefully avoided providing numerical indices to differentiate severity (e.g., in the sleep-related breathing disorders). This was done because a single numerical cut point (such as the apnea index) is often not an appropriate division between levels of severity, and clinical judgment of several indices of severity is considered superior. Additional clinical information contained in the severity criteria indicates to the clinician which parameters should be considered in deciding the severity of the disorder.
>
> It is emphasized that these criteria are a guide, are not absolute, and are to be applied in conjunction with consideration of the patient's clinical status.[52(p. 22)]

Methodological Concerns

- Severity categories may be arbitrary and unrelated to meaningful outcome measures.
- The evaluation of large numbers of particularly "severe" patients with high RDIs, impressive hypoxemia, sleep fragmentation, excessive daytime sleepiness, hypertension, and cardiac arrhythmias may produce a type of medical "grade inflation," where patients with less severe findings may not be deemed to have clinically significant findings. Labeling a patient disorder "mild" may result in the false impression that the patient does not have a clinically significant disorder. This in turn can result in denial of treatment or insurance coverage for recommended treatment.
- Most published severity rating systems depend primarily on the RDI and do not specify cutoffs for other important polysomnographic data, such as hypoxia, or specify which cardiac arrhythmias may require a change in rating category.

Existing Definitions

- *International Classification of Sleep Disorders.*[52] As noted previously, this classification system avoided providing specific numerical cutoffs for RDI, SaO_2, and specification of cardiac arrhythmias. However, it does provide a general set of guidelines that can be followed by the interpreter:

  Mild: The majority of the habitual sleep period is free of respiratory disturbance. The apneic episodes are associated with mild oxygen desaturation or benign cardiac arrhythmias. A mild disorder is associated with mild sleepiness or mild insomnia.

  Moderate: A moderate disorder can be associated with moderate oxygen desaturation or mild cardiac arrhythmias. It is associated with moderate sleepiness or mild insomnia.

  Severe: The majority of the habitual sleep period is associated with respiratory disturbance, with severe oxygen desaturation or moderate to severe cardiac arrhythmias. Evidence might be found of associated cardiac or pulmonary failure. A severe disorder is associated with severe sleepiness.

- *American Academy of Sleep Medicine Task Force on Sleep-Related Breathing Disorders in Adults.*[29] The task force noted that severity of the obstructive sleep apnea should be based on two components: the polysomnogram and daytime sleepiness. The task force based its breakdown of severity on polysomnographically derived event frequency (RDI) taken from Wisconsin Sleep Cohort data.[58] These data demonstrated an increased risk of hypertension that becomes highly significant when the RDI is ≥30/hr of sleep. The task force stated that currently no data are available to indicate where the distinction between mild and moderate degrees of sleep-disordered breathing should be drawn. The task force recommendation of an RDI of 15/hr of sleep was based on a consensus of task force members' opinions:

  Mild: 5–15 events/hr.

  Moderate: 15–30 events/hr.

  Severe: >30 events/hr.

- *American Sleep Disorders Association Practice Parameters for the Treatment of OSA in Adults.*[59] Although this was not published to provide guidelines for determining diagnostic severity, it does consider what level of severity is necessary to justify treatment with CPAP:

  An apnea index of at least 20/hr or an apnea/hypopnea index of at least 30/hr, regardless of the patient's symptoms.

  AHI of at least 10/hr in a patient with excessive daytime sleepiness.

A respiratory arousal index of at least 10/hr in a patient with excessive daytime sleepiness.

Figure 4-7 shows a compressed 4 min portion of the diagnostic PSG of a 43-year-old man presenting for evaluation of possible sleep apnea. Overall RDI was only 9.0/hr of sleep and 14/hr of sleep during REM sleep. The obstructive apnea seen in the figure lasted 110 sec and was associated with a low SaO$_2$, which read 2%. As noted in the SaO$_2$ section, it is unlikely that this SaO$_2$ value is real, but it is clear that the low SaO$_2$ is well below 50%. This apnea was associated with decrease in heart rate from 85 to 60 BPM, but otherwise no cardiac arrhythmias were noted. Although the overall RDI is most consistent with mild obstructive sleep apnea, due to the severe hypoxemia, it was read as severe.

The change in severity ratings from mild to severe based on the single apnea shown in Figure 4-7 is understandable. However, there are no generally accepted specific cutoffs for evaluating the clinical significance of milder levels of hypoxemia.

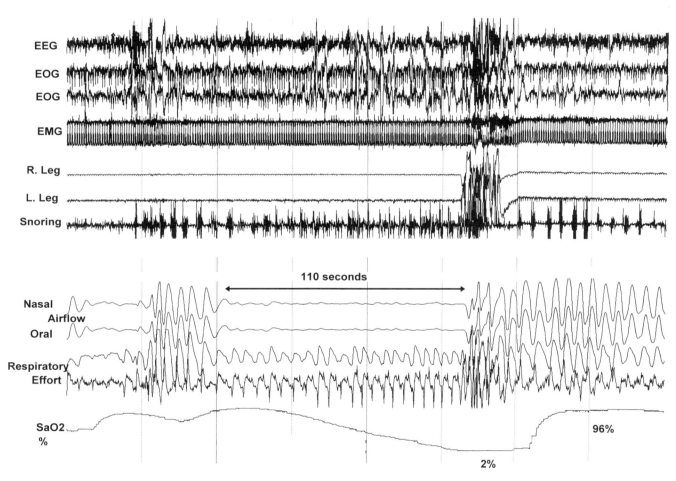

FIGURE 4-7
Effects of severe hypoxia on severity statements.

5

Evaluation of Movement-Related Data

Measurement of limb movements is an essential part of diagnostic polysomnography. The diagnosis of periodic leg movements in sleep, restless legs syndrome, and REM behavior disorder all depend of the acquisition and interpretation of movement-related data.

GENERAL ALGORITHM FOR INTERPRETATION OF MOVEMENT DATA

For movements consistent with periodic leg movement in sleep (PLMS),

1. Identify movement or EMG variables recorded.
2. Identify the method of recording (EMG vs. movement).
3. Specify working definitions for different types of movements (arousing vs. nonarousing).
4. Review raw polysomnogram (PSG) recording and verify movement episodes have been scored according to predetermined sleep laboratory procedures.
5. Review raw PSG recording and verify movement episodes identified as periodic leg movements are not movements occurring in association with general arousals or general body movements of the type often seen at the termination of apneas or hypopneas.
6. Examine summary data.
7. Examine histograms to permit correlation of PLMS with changes in sleep and other parameters.

THE MAJORITY OF THE EPOCH RULE AND SCORING OF MOVEMENTS IN SLEEP

The majority of the epoch (MOE) rule does not apply directly to the analysis of movement data. However, it has a direct effect on the computation of indexes such as the periodic leg movements in sleep index (PLMSI) and arousing periodic leg movements in sleep index (APLMSI), which are based on the number of episodes per hour of scored sleep. Leg movements may occur during epochs scored as sleep or wakefulness. Some scorers and interpreters, as well as many automated and semiautomated systems, may not include scored leg movements in summary data if they were noted during epochs scored as wake. In the typical 30 sec scoring epoch, wake may consist of 16 sec and sleep, 14 sec. As the MOE rule requires that the epoch be scored according to the sleep state (or wake) that occupies the majority of the epoch, significant amounts of sleep and potentially frequent leg movements can be eliminated from the final summary. This can lead to a dramatic reduction in scored PLMSI or APLMSI that does not reflect the actual severity of movement-related sleep disorders in the sleep recording.

ABBREVIATIONS OF TERMINOLOGY

PLMS (periodic leg movements in sleep or periodic limb movements in sleep).
APLMS (arousing periodic leg movements in sleep or arousing periodic limb movements in sleep).

PERIODIC LEG MOVEMENTS IN SLEEP

Definition

As originally defined by Coleman,[60] periodic leg movements in sleep are bursts of EMG activity measured at the anterior tibialis muscle lasting 0.5–5 sec and repeating every 4–90 sec with at least four movements during behavioral sleep. These occur almost exclusively during non-REM (NREM) sleep.

General Significance

A potential source of sleep fragmentation resulting in complaints of daytime sleepiness, frequent awakenings from sleep and nonrestorative sleep. Increases in frequency with age.

Alternative Terminology

PLMS also is called *nocturnal myoclonus* and *periodic limb movements in sleep*.

Methodological Concerns

Arousing versus Nonarousing Periodic Leg Movements in Sleep

PLMS not associated with EEG-defined arousal sometimes are thought not to be of clinical significance. However, the determination of whether a PLMS is arousing or nonarousing depends on how arousal is measured. It has been noted that in the absence of traditionally defined EEG arousal PLMS still may be associated with so-called autonomic arousal—specifically, changes in blood pressure and heart rate (Figure 5-1). The clinical significance of these findings and its contribution to the patient's sleep/wake complaints is uncertain.

Arousal Threshold

Another factor difficult to assess is the arousal threshold. The sleep fragmentation literature notes that, as sleep fragmentation continues, the same stimuli have a harder time producing arousal. Applied to the question of arousing vs. nonarousing PLMS, the arousal threshold may be a controlling factor. The higher the arousing threshold, the less likely that PLMS will cause arousal. Therefore, it may be wise to consider all nonarousing PLMS as potentially arousing and potentially clinically significant under certain conditions.

Mixtures of Leg Movements and Episodes of Sleep-Disordered Breathing

When leg movements and sleep-disordered breathing appear concurrently, the interpreter ultimately must be responsible for determining which is primary and which is secondary. A leg movement (or increase in anterior tibialis EMG) occurring during the general arousal complex that typically occurs at the termination of apneas and hypopnea most likely does not represent a movement associated with the independently occurring sleep-disorder PLMS. Alternately, changes in respiration occurring after a leg or body movement may represent an artifact and not an apnea or hypopnea as usually defined.

Minimal Number of Repetitive Movements and Arousal

As noted in the definition, PLMS is a disorder of repetitive movements. A minimum of four consecutive movements must be noted. In practice, however, PLMS can result in arousal or even complete awakening from sleep that may limit the number of repetitive leg movements.

FACTORS OR MEDICAL CONDITIONS ASSOCIATED WITH INCREASED PERIODIC LEG MOVEMENTS IN SLEEP

- Absence of frequent episodes of sleep-disordered breathing.
- Older age.
- Tricyclic antidepressants.
- Withdrawal from central nervous system (CNS) depressants and sedatives or hypnotics that suppress PLMS.
- End-stage renal failure and dialysis.
- Anemia.
- Decreased percentage or quantity of REM sleep.

FACTORS OR MEDICAL CONDITIONS ASSOCIATED WITH DECREASED PERIODIC LEG MOVEMENTS IN SLEEP

- Medication:
  Benzodiazepines.
  Dopamine agonists.
  Other CNS depressants.
- Sleep severely fragmented by sleep-disordered breathing.
- Increased percentage or quantity of REM sleep.

Severity

There are no experimentally validated classification systems for determining severity of PLMS.

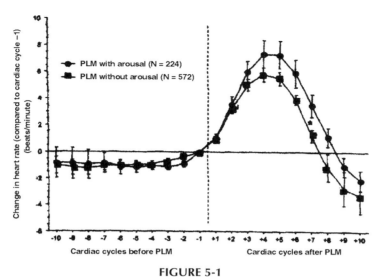

FIGURE 5-1

PLMS and evoked heart rate. (Reprinted with permission from Winkleman J. Heart rate response to periodic leg movements of sleep. *Sleep.* 1999;22:576–580.)

Existing Classifications

International Classification of Sleep Disorders[52]

Mild: PLM index of 5 or more but less than 25, mild insomnia or mild sleepiness.

Moderate: PLM index of 25 or more but less than 50, moderate insomnia or moderate sleepiness.

Severe: PLM index of 50 or more or a PLM-arousal index of greater than 25, severe insomnia or sleepiness.

As most of the clinical symptoms of PLMS appear to be a result of sleep fragmentation, it of interest that the International Classification of Sleep Disorders does not provide PLMS arousal index cutoffs for mild and moderate PLMS. It seems reasonable for the interpreter to also rely on general findings regarding the consequences of experimental sleep fragmentation (see Table 2-2), changes associated with different respiratory disturbance index levels (at lower RDIs, hypoxemia may be presumed to be less of a factor) and the nocturnal determinants of daytime sleepiness (see Table 6-1).

Figure 5-1 presents a comparison of changes in heart rate immediately following PLMS associated with American Sleep Disorders Association (ASDA)-defined EEG arousal and without EEG arousal. An evoked heart rate suggesting autonomic arousal is present both with and without EEG arousal. A similar experimental report using tones to produce changes in blood pressure or heart rate without EEG arousal found a significant decrease in mean sleep latency on the MSLT (see Table 2-2).

6

Objective Measurement of Daytime Sleepiness

MULTIPLE SLEEP LATENCY TEST

Definition

The Multiple Sleep Latency Test (MSLT) is the generally accepted objective measure of daytime sleepiness. It is based on the simple principle that sleepy individuals will fall asleep faster than more alert individuals.

General Significance

Patients presenting with sleep complaints may deny or actually be unaware of the presence or severity of their daytime sleepiness. Even those patients who actually fall asleep during office consultations or in the waiting room may report themselves as alert. Patients may lose an appropriate "frame of reference" as to how alert they actually are compared to others after only a few weeks of partial sleep deprivation or hypnotic or sedative drug use. For this reason, a technique not dependent on the patient's subjective report of alertness was necessary. The MSLT was created to fulfill this need.

General Methodology

The generally accepted and endorsed methodology for conducting the MSLT (Table 6-1) should be followed exactly to avoid problems. Failure to strictly follow this routine increases the risk of false negative and positive findings. Sleep technologists should document this routine carefully, and the interpreter should review these documents prior to making any final statements about the MSLT.

Methodological Concerns

- Daytime alertness and sleepiness are very sensitive to the quantity and quality of not only the prior night's sleep but reductions or extensions in typical sleep over days, weeks, or longer (Figure 6-1). One or two nights of reduced sleep time or sleep fragmentation on the nights prior to testing may result in significant changes in sleep latencies, interpretation, and final diagnosis.
- Daytime alertness may be susceptible to the effects of a wide variety of medications.

TABLE 6-1
Procedures Prior to Start of MSLT

Time	Procedure
30 min prior to testing	Suspend tobacco smoking
15 min prior to testing	Suspend vigorous physical exercise
10 min prior to testing	Prepare for bed: Remove shoes Loosen constricting clothing
5 min prior to testing	In bed, hooked up: Calibrations
45 sec prior to testing	Introspective sleepiness measure
30 sec prior to testing	Assume comfortable position for falling asleep
5 sec prior to testing	"Please lie quietly, keep your eyes closed, and try to fall asleep"

Source: Modified from Carskadon MA, Dement WC, Mitler MM, Roth T, Westbrook PR, Keenan S. Guidelines for the multiple sleep latency test (MSLT): A standard measure of sleepiness. *Sleep*. 1986; 9(4):519–524.

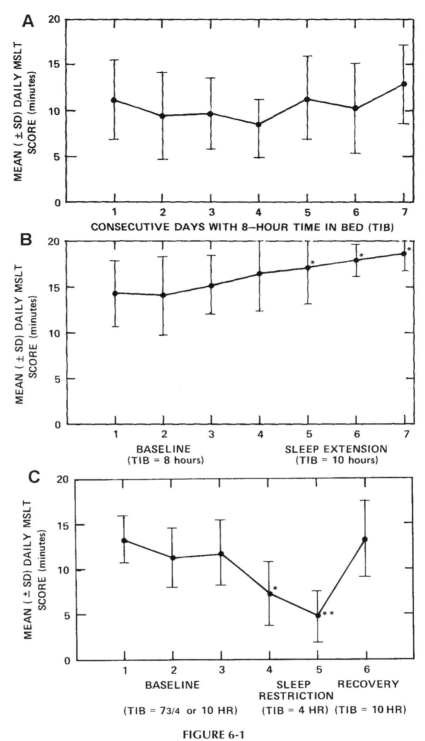

FIGURE 6-1

Determinants of daytime sleepiness. **(A)** Stability of MSLT scores for a group of young adults (mean age 20.2 yr, range 18–23 yr) who kept to a fixed sleep schedule of 8 hr for seven consecutive days. **(B)** Effects of sleep extension on young adults (mean age 19 yr, range 18–20 yr). Subjects kept to a fixed 8 hr schedule for first three nights and then increased time in bed to 10 hours by advancing lights out to 10 PM. Total sleep time increased from 437 ± 23 min to 510 ± 44 min between the two conditions. Although the mean sleep latency during the 8 hr condition had been around 15 min—consistent with normal alertness—the mean sleep latency increased further to 19 min with sleep extension. Values were statistically different from baseline starting with first night of sleep extension. **(C)** Effects of acute sleep restriction on eight young adults (mean age 20.7 yr, range 17–25 yr). A single night in which sleep is reduced from 10 hr, or 7.75 hr, to 4 hr was sufficient to reduce the mean sleep latency to <5 min for three subjects after only one night and, in the remaining subjects, after two nights. This finding strongly suggests that the MSLT is very sensitive to reductions in usual sleep time. A single bad night in the sleep laboratory prior to the MSLT could result in a finding of severe daytime sleepiness vs. normal alertness. For this reason, all MSLTs must be preceded by an all-night polysomnogram.

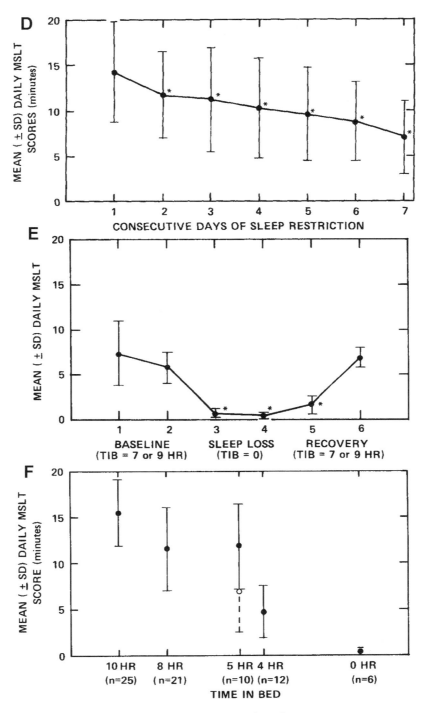

FIGURE 6-1 *continued*

(D) Effects of partial cumulative sleep deprivation on young adults (mean age 20.0 yr, range 17–24 yr) over seven nights. Following three nights restricted to 10 hr in bed, subjects were restricted to 5 hr in bed. By the end of the seven nights, 50% of subjects had mean sleep latency of <5 min and all but one of the remaining subjects had sleep latencies in the 5–10 min range. A single subject maintained a mean sleep latency of >10 min throughout the study. **(E)** Effects of total sleep deprivation on young adults (mean age 19.2 yr, range 18–21 yr). After one night of total sleep deprivation, mean sleep latency fell to almost 0.0 min. Subjects slept their habitual amount prior to sleep deprivation and may have been partially sleep deprived. **(F)** Average of mean daily MSLT scores for each of the groups in plots A–E. (Reprinted with permission from Carskadon MA, Dement WC. Nocturnal determinants of daytime sleepiness. *Sleep.* 1982;5(2)(Suppl):S73–81.)

The MSLT interpreter therefore must have access to data from the following before any interpretation can be done:

Data from a full polysomnogram (PSG) conducted on the night before the MSLT.
Data from a sleep log for at least one week prior to the MSLT.
A full accounting of medications, especially those that might affect daytime alertness.

- MSLT findings may not be directly relevant to daytime performance of the patient. The interpreter should be very careful to interpret only the MSLT finding and not make predictions about future patient behavior.
- The MSLT also is very susceptible to disruption from many sources during data acquisition. Any behavior or occurrence that causes the patient to become activated could result in a delay in sleep latency and change in mean sleep latency. Factors that could delay sleep onset include:
  Physical exertion, even an undemanding walk.
  Social interaction, an offhand remark by the technologist just prior to lights out has been known to result in delayed sleep onset or no sleep at all in the allotted time.
  Discussion of results of PSG from the prior night.
  Caffeine.
  Nicotine.
  Noise.
  Uncomfortable bed or pillow.
  Routine medication.
  Timing or type of meals, snacks, or drinks.
  Doing anything atypical for the patient.
  Testing anxiety.
  "Cabin fever" after extended testing.

Figure 6-2 shows the results of MSLT across the day with each nap preceded by a 5 min walk or 5 min TV watching. Testing was performed after a typical night of sleep and after a night of partial sleep deprivation. Following typical nights of sleep, the mean sleep latency following the 5 min walk was 13.6 ± 5.2 compared to 6.7 ± 5.2 min following TV watching.

EXISTING DEFINITIONS OF DAYTIME SLEEPINESS SEVERITY

The following definitions are modified from the International Classification of Sleep Disorders:[52]

Mild sleepiness: Mean sleep latency of 10–15 min. This term describes sleep episodes that are present only during times of rest or when little attention is required. Situations in which mild sleepiness can become evident include but are not limited to lying down in a quiet room, watching television, reading, or being a passenger in a moving vehicle. Mild sleepiness may not be present every day. The symptoms of mild sleepiness produce a minor impairment of social or occupational function.
Moderate sleepiness: Mean sleep latency of 5–10 min. This term describes sleep episodes that are present daily and that occur during very mild physical activities requiring, at most, a moderate degree of attention. Examples of situations in which moderate sleepiness may occur include driving and attending concerts, theater, or similar group meetings. The symptoms of moderate sleepiness produce a moderate impairment of social or occupational function.
Severe sleepiness: Mean sleep latency of less than 5 min. This term describes sleep episodes that are present daily and at times of physical activities that require mild to moderate attention. Examples of situations in which severe sleepiness may occur include eating, direct personal conversation, driving, walking, and physical activities. The symptoms of severe sleepi-

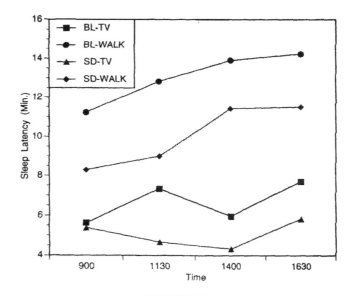

FIGURE 6-2

MSLT problems. (Reprinted with permission from Bonnet MH, Arand DL. Sleepiness measured by modified multiple sleep latency testing varies as a function of preceding activity. *Sleep.* 1998;21(50):477–483.)

ness produce a marked impairment of social or occupational function.

These categories are somewhat general. The interpreter may want to further identify what groups of patients or experimental subjects have shown similar mean MSLT latencies for points of comparison. Table 6-2 lists more than 60 published research studies that used the MSLT.

SLEEP-ONSET REM PERIODS

In addition to the measurement of daytime sleepiness, the MSLT plays an important role in providing objective support for the diagnosis of narcolepsy. In normal individuals, REM sleep generally occurs 90–120 min after sleep onset. However, in many patients with nar-

colepsy, REM sleep will occur within 15 min of sleep onset. This early period of REM sleep, called a *sleep-onset REM period* (SOREMP), under certain conditions is considered objective support for the diagnosis of narcolepsy. The usual requirement is that SOREMPs must be noted on at least two of the five nap opportunities of the MSLT. The threshold of at least two SOREMPs was set with the understanding that occasionally SOREMPs might appear in patients who do not have narcolepsy. However, it has more recently become clear that two or more SOREMPS may occur in a variety of patients without narcolepsy as well as asymptomatic research subjects during a standard MSLT. The data reported in Table 6-3 are the results of a retrospective review of more than 2,000 MSLTs for the presence of SOREMPs.[85] Two or more SOREMPs were noted for 80% of the patients with narcolepsy and 6.6% of nonnarcoleptic subjects.

TABLE 6-2
MSLT Results by Group

Mean Sleep Latency (min)	Standard Deviation or Range	Sleep-Onset REM Periods	Description	Reference
2.2	1.9		Elderly normals after 38 hr total sleep deprivation $N = 10$, 2 men, 8 women, mean age 69.3 yr	61
2.5	1.5	3.6	Narcoleptics, $N = 11$, 4 men, 7 women, age 39.4 yr, drug free = 2 weeks	62
2.6	1.7		OSA, $N = 10$, 9 men, 1 woman, mean age 50.5 yr, SL = 1 epoch, RDI = 28–91/hr	61
2.6	3.1	3.7/pt	Narcolepsy, $N = 20$, 10 men, 10 women, mean age 47 yr, up to 30 mg methylphenidate permitted	63
2.8	?		Narcoleptics, $N = 19$, 12 men, 7 women, mean age 44.9 yr, drug free 1 week, SL = 1 epoch	64
2.8	2.1	3.4/pt	Narcoleptics following GHB administration hs for 29 days, $N = 20$, 10 men, 10 women, mean age 47 yr, up to 30 mg methylphenidate permitted (no different from baseline, 2.6 vs. 2.8)	63
3.0	*	72%	Narcolepsy, $N = 50$, 27 men, 23 women, mean age 42 yr	65
3.2	*	10%	OSA, AI >30/hr, $N = 41$, 40 men, 1 woman, mean age 47 yr	66
3.3	3.3		Narcoleptics	67
3.3	0.3	54%	Narcoleptics, $N = 222$, 125 men, 97 women, mean age ~45 yr, 5 yr retrospective case series of clinical patients, drug free = 2 weeks, SL = 1 epoch	68
4.3	1.2	20%	Narcolepsy, $N = 10$, 6 men, 4 women, mean age 44.2 yr	69
4.6		3.1/pt	Narcolepsy, $N = 66$, 34 men, 32 women, mean age 45.4 yr, drug free = ?, SL = 1 epoch	70
4.7	?		OSA, post-UPPP, $N = 5$, 5 men, mean age ~50 yr, RDI decreased from 66.5 to 38.2/hr, mean MSLT increased from 3.2 to 4.7 min	63
4.7	1.9–6.8	0	Idiopathic CNS hypersomnolence?, $N = 11$, 6 men, 5 women, mean age 40.8 yr, SL = ?, drug free = 30 days	71
5.1	0.57		Idiopathic CNS hypersomnolence, $N = 34$, 18 men, 16 women, mean age ~44 yr, drug free = 2 weeks	68
5.2	0.75		Narcoleptics, $N = 15$, mean age 32 yr, SL = ?, untreated/drug free	72

continues

TABLE 6-2   *continued*
MSLT Results by Group

Mean Sleep Latency (min)	Standard Deviation or Range	Sleep-Onset REM Periods	Description	Reference
5.3			OSA, $N = 9$, 8 men, 1 woman, mean age 49.9 yr, no RDI reported, no meds 2 weeks, SL = 3 epochs	73
5.8		0.4/pt	Insufficient sleep, cc = EDS, $N = 59$, 37 men, 22 women, mean age 40.8 yr, SL = 1 epoch, prior night TST 501 min, patients reported usual sleep at home 6.2 hr, TST at home suggests chronic partial sleep deprivation of ~2.2 hr/night, results of 1 night with 8.4 hr TST	70
6.0	*	8%	Insufficient sleep, $N = 23$, 12 men, 11 women, mean age 42 yr, prior TST = 495 min	66
6.1	0.82		Narcoleptics, $N = 32$, 23 men, 9 women, mean age 40.5 yr, drug free = 2 weeks, SL = ?, after 33 hr ad lib sleeping	72
6.6			Narcoleptics, $N = 12$, 9 men, 3 women, mean age 41.8 yr, no meds 2 weeks, st 1 lat, requires 3 epochs	73
6.9	*	18%	Periodic leg movements in sleep, $N = 12$, 8 men, 4 women, mean age 51 yr	66
6.9	4.5		Chronic insomnia treated with 15 mg flurazepam, $N = 6$, 1 man, 5 women, age 67–72 yr, alertness decreased compared to placebo MSLT (9.8 vs. 6.9 min)	74
7.5		?	Normal controls following 5 hr prior nocturnal sleep and administration of ethanol (0.75 g/kg) at 9:30 AM before MSLT, $N = 18$, mean age 25.6 yr	75
7.7	3.9	?	EDS complaint, majority OSA, $N = 29$, 16 men, 13 women, mean age 50.2 yr, mean RDI = 39.5	76
8.3			Normal controls following 8 hr prior nocturnal sleep and administration of ethanol (0.75 g/kg) at 9:30 AM before MSLT, $N = 18$, mean age 25.6 yr	75
8.5			Insomnia treated with 30 mg flurazepam, $N = 23$, 10 men, 13 women, mean age 37 yr, SL = ?, mean of two 6 nap MSLTs on consecutive days, highly variable latencies (decreased alertness from baseline, MSLT 12.8 to 8.5 min)	77
8.6			Misc. EDS (not narcolepsy or OSA) $N = 14$, no meds 2 weeks, st 1 lat, requires 3 epochs	74
9.0	4.9		Psychiatric patients	67
9.0	*		Normals with a mean screening MSLT latency ≤6 min after 3 nights of sleep extension to 10 hr, $N = 12$, 12 men, mean age 25.2 yr, drug free, SL = 1 epoch, prior estimated TST = 7 hr	78
9.8	4.4		Chronic insomnia treated with placebo, $N = 6$, 1 man, 5 women, ages 67–72 yr	74
9.9	?		Normals, $N = 5$, 2 men, 3 women, mean age 30 yr, prior night's TST not reported	65
10.0			Primary depression, $N = 7$, 2 men, 5 women, mean age 37.1 yr, no meds 2 weeks, SL = 3 epochs	73
10.3	4.2	?	Normals, $N = 10$, 2 men, 8 women, mean age 69.3 yr, first recovery night after 38 hr total sleep deprivation, TST = 531 min	61
10.5	*	8%	Psychiatric, $N = 13$, 4 men, 9 women, mean age 44 yr	66
10.9	5.0		Normal sleepers, $N = 89$, 49 men, 40 women, age 26.5 yr, drug free = 2 weeks, SL = 1 epoch, prior night's sleep = 449 min	79
11.0	*		Normals with a mean screening MSLT latency ≤6 min, after 6 nights' sleep extension to 10 hr, $N = 12$, 12 men, age 25.2 yr, drug free, SL = 1 epoch, prior estimated TST = 7 hr	78
11.1	5.5	0%	Normals, $N = 8$, 4 men, 4 women, mean age 44.6 yr, drug free = 3 months	69
11.3			Normal controls following 11 hr prior nocturnal sleep and administration of ethanol (0.75 g/kg) at 9:30 AM before MSLT, $N = 18$, mean age 25.6 yr	75
12.1	3.2		Normals characterized as evening types (Owls) by Horne and Ostberg questionnaire, $N = 10$, age 19–28 yr, not different from morning types (Larks) (MSLT 12.1 vs. 12.9 min)	80

continues

TABLE 6-2 *continued*

MSLT Results by Group

Mean Sleep Latency (min)	Standard Deviation or Range	Sleep-Onset REM Periods	Description	Reference
12.2			Chronic insomniacs, $N = 25$, 8 men, 17 women, mean age 69.6 yr, drug free, prior night TST = 400 min	81
12.2	4.4	?	Normals, $N = 10$, 2 men, 8 women, mean age 69.3 yr, after 7.7 hr TST, arousal index = 10.3	61
12.2			Normals, $N = 45$, 31 men, 14 women, mean age 50.4 yr, drug free = ?, SL = 1 epoch, mean prior night's TST = 419 min	82
12.4	5.4	?	Chronic insomniacs, $N = 138$, 43 men, 95 women, mean age 55 yr, prior night TST = 401 min	79
12.8	2.5–18		Insomnia, $N = 23$, 10 men, 13 women, mean age 37 yr, drug free = 7 days, SL = ?, mean of two 6-nap MSLTs on consecutive days, highly variable latencies	77
12.8	1.4		Normals characterized as morning types (Larks) by Horne and Ostberg questionnaire, $N = 8$, age 19–28 yr, no different from evening types (Owls) (MSLT 12.9 vs. 12.1 min)	80
12.9	7.9		Normals, $N = 10$, approx age 50 yr, SL = first epoch, prior night TST = 410 min	63
13.0	*	5%	EDS, no PSG findings, $N = 22$, 10 men, 12 women, mean age 32 yr	66
13.3	4.6		Chronic insomniacs treated with 0.25 mg placebo, $N = 7$, 3 men, 4 women, age 64–79 yr	74
13.4			Chronic insomniacs, $N = 50$, 20 men, 30 women, mean age 44.3 yr, drug free, prior night TST = 375 min	82
13.6	4.5	?	Normals, $N = 10$, 2 men, 8 women, mean age 69.3 yr, second recovery night after 38 hr total sleep deprivation, TST = 437 min	61
13.8	2.6		Normals after 24 hr sleep deprivation followed by a 1 hr nap, $N = 40$, 20 men, 20 women, ages 18-35 yr	81
14.4	5.6–18.4		Insomnia treated with 0.5 mg triazolam, $N = 23$, 10 men, 13 women, mean age 37 yr, SL = ?, mean of two 6 nap MSLTs on consecutive days, highly variable latencies (increased alertness from baseline MSLT 12.8 to 14.4 min)	77
14.7			Chronic insomnia, $N = 70$, 37 men, 33 women, mean age 47.8 yr, drug free = ?, SL = 1 epoch, mean prior night's TST = 364 min	82
15.0	3.7	0.1	Normal, $N = 11$, 4 men, 7 women, mean age 39.4 yr, drug free	62
15.1			Normal controls following 5 hr prior nocturnal sleep and administration of caffeine (4 mg/kg) at 9:30 AM before MSLT, $N = 18$, mean age 25.6 yr	75
15.9			Normal controls following 8 hr prior nocturnal sleep and administration of caffeine (4 mg/kg) at 9:30 AM before MSLT, $N = 18$, mean age 25.6 yr	75
16.9			Normal controls following 11 hr prior nocturnal sleep and administration of caffeine (4 mg/kg) at 9:30 AM before MSLT, $N = 18$, mean age 25.6 yr	75
16.9	3.6		Chronic insomnia treated with 0.25 mg triazolam, $N = 7$, 3 men, 4 women, age 64–79 yr, alertness improved compared to placebo, MSLT (13.3 vs. 16.9 min)	74
17.5	*		Normals with a mean screening MSLT latency ≥16 min, after 3 nights' sleep extension to 10 hr, $N = 12$, 12 men, aged 23.8 yr, drug free, SL = 1 epoch, prior estimated TST = 7.6 hr	78
18.0	*		Normals with a mean screening MSLT latency ≥16 min, after 6 nights' sleep extension to 10 hr, $N = 12$, 12 men, aged 23.8 yr, drug free, SL = 1 epoch, prior estimated TST = 7.6 hr	78
26.4	2.8	0	Normal children, $N = 18$, 9 boys, 9 girls, age 8–12 yr, 30 min allowed for each nap instead of usual 20 min, 5 children failed to fall asleep at all, only one third of children fell asleep on each nap	84

Note: This is a listing of sleep research studies by descending mean sleep latency with a brief description of patient group or experimental procedure. Where available, the number of sleep-onset REM periods (SOREMPs) noted are presented.

Abbreviations: pt = patients, OSA = obstructive sleep apnea, SL = sleep latency, RDI = respiratory disturbance index, GHB = gammahydroxybutyrate, AI = apnea index, UPPP = uvula palatopharyngoplasty, CNS = central nervous system, cc = chief complaint, EDS = excessive daytime sleepiness, TST = total sleep time, st 1 lat = stage 1 latency, ? = unknown.

*Estimated.

TABLE 6-3
Sleep-Onset REM Periods in Narcoleptics and Nonnarcoleptics

	Narcolepsy with Cataplexy	Narcolepsy without Cataplexy	Sleep-Related Breathing Disorders	Other Sleep Disorders
N	106	64	1,251	662
0 SOREMPs	13%	3%	84%	82%
1 SOREMPs	13%	6%	9%	11%
2 SOREMPs	24%	45%	5%	5%
3 SOREMPs	26%	28%	1%	1.2%
4–5 SOREMPs	24%	17%	0.3%	0.5%
2 or more SOREMPs	74%	91%	7%	7%
Mean sleep latency <5 min	87%	81%	39%	23%
Mean sleep latency <8 min	93%	97%	63%	48%
>2 SOREMPs + mean sleep latency <5 min	67%	75%	4%	1.5%
>2 SOREMPs + mean sleep latency <8 min	71%	91%	6%	4%*
SOREMP on polysomnogram	33%	24%	1%	1.7%

*13 of 27 with possible narcolepsy.

Source: Reprinted with permission from Aldrich MS, Chervin RD, Malow B. Value of the multiple sleep latency test for the diagnosis of narcolepsy. *Sleep*. 1997;20(8):620–629.

Additional studies of multiple SOREMPs during MSLT testing with nonnarcoleptics report the following:

- In normal adolescents, 4 of 26 students in the 10th grade (mean age 15 yr) had two or more SOREMPs and another 7 had a single SOREMP. All SOREMPs occurred during the first two nap opportunities of the day, at 8:30 AM and 10:30 AM. This suggests that these SOREMPs occurred secondary to a combination of both a phase delay in the student sleep/wake rhythms and the early rise time required to get to school on time. Therefore, these students underwent testing during a time when their circadian systems (based on body temperature) had a high likelihood of initiating REM sleep[14] (see Figure 2-5).
- In normal controls (mean age 27.9 ± 9.5 yr) screened for participation in sleep research projects, of the 139 subjects tested, 24 (17%) showed ≥2 SOREMPs.

Those subjects with SOREMPs also were sleepier than subjects without SOREMPs (mean sleep latency 6.2 ± 2.9 vs. 10.8 ± 4.5 min), leading to the suspicion that these SOREMPs might be secondary to the effects of chronic insufficient sleep.[86]

Multiple SOREMPs on the MSLT occur much more frequently in patients with narcolepsy than patients without narcolepsy. However, the rate of multiple SOREMPs in nonnarcoleptics is sufficiently high that SOREMPs cannot be used as an independent diagnostic marker for narcolepsy. The significance of SOREMPs cannot be understood in a vacuum. SOREMPs should not be used to make a diagnosis of narcolepsy in the absence of a consistent clinical history, preferably with auxiliary symptoms, and with a prior night's PSG to rule out the possibility of other sleep disorders.

7

Introduction to Continuous/Bilevel Positive Airway Pressure Treatment Trials and Split Night Studies

CONTINUOUS POSITIVE AIRWAY PRESSURE

Definition

Administration of continuous positive airway pressure (CPAP) generally is considered the state of the art treatment for moderate and severe obstructive sleep apnea. CPAP administration requires titration or dosing of different pressure levels to determine the optimal pressure. Typically, the polysomnogram (PSG) technician on duty monitors the patient's ongoing sleep and respiration, making adjustments to pressure levels until optimal reduction in sleep-disordered breathing and optimal improvement in sleep quantity and quality is reached. Generally, this pressure will then be set on the home nasal continuous positive airway pressure (NCPAP) machine the patient is expected to use thereafter on a nightly basis. Although many attempts to predict the optimal pressure for a particular patient without in-laboratory titration have been published, none has proven as successful as classic sleep laboratory CPAP titration.

General Significance

Generally, only a single night in the sleep laboratory is permitted to complete titration and identify the optimal treatment for the patient.

General Methodology

During a full polysomnogram:

- Reduce episodes of sleep-disordered breathing, sleep fragmentation, hypoxemia, cardiac arrhythmias, and snoring to the lowest level possible.

- Administer the lowest positive airway pressure possible.
- Ensure that the patient not only tolerates the treatment but feels sufficiently comfortable to consider home NCPAP therapy.

Methodological Concerns

The success or failure of an NCPAP treatment trial depends on a wide variety of factors, many of which are not under the direct control of the sleep specialist or sleep technologist. The following factors contribute to a successful NCPAP treatment trial:

- Patient spends sufficient time in bed.
- Patient sleeps sufficient quantity.
- Patient sleeps in supine position.
- Patient sleeps in a supine position early in the recording to allow sufficient time to titrate the pressure.
- REM sleep is present in sufficient quantities.
- REM sleep is present early in recording to allow sufficient time to titrate the pressure.
- Patient falls asleep quickly, once NCPAP mask is positioned and positive pressure started.
- Patient tolerates CPAP mask and pressures.
- Patient is not aroused by increasing pressure levels during titration.
- Patient is able to breathe nasally.
- Patient does not develop side effects:
  Dry mouth.
  Nasal congestion.
  Facial pain.
  Headache.
  Claustrophobia.

• Technical staff is sufficiently sophisticated, trained, and alert to properly titrate pressures and respond to problems as they occur.

These factors contribute to failure:

• NCPAP titration requires administration of numerous pressure levels.
• The highest level of NCPAP pressure administered is insufficient to reduce the respiratory disturbance index (RDI) to expected levels.
• Optimal reduction in sleep-disordered breathing may not occur due to insufficient sleep time.
• Apneas and hypopneas are present primarily during REM sleep or in a supine position.
• Patient does not spend sufficient time in REM sleep in a supine position.
• REM sleep is absent.
• Patient does not or will not sleep in supine position.
• Patient spends insufficient time in bed.
• Patient sleeps insufficient quantity.
• Patient is unable to tolerate CPAP mask and pressures.
• Patient refuses to permit increase in pressure levels.
• Patient is unable to breathe nasally.
• Patient develops side effects:
  Dry mouth.
  Nasal congestion.
  Facial pain.
  Headache.
  Claustrophobia.
• Patient removes CPAP mask and refuses to continue treatment trial.
• Patient removes CPAP mask as well as electrodes and sensors and leaves sleep laboratory before titration complete.
• Technical staff is not sufficiently sophisticated, trained, and alert to titrate pressures or respond to problems as they occur.

Identifying Optimal Pressure Level

The interpreter should consider each period during which a different positive airway pressure is administered as if it were a separate polysomnogram. Sleep and respiratory data at each pressure level should be separately evaluated for

• RDI, SaO_2, snoring, cardiac arrhythmias, sleep quantity, and quality.
• The presence of factors, such as a supine position and REM sleep, that would define a period of highest risk for obstructive sleep apnea and its associated findings. The effectiveness of CPAP easily can

be underestimated if the lowest RDI occurs during a period when REM sleep or a supine position is not present. For example,

As seen in Table 7-1, based on the lowest RDI, a pressure of 10 cm H_2O would have been determined to be optimal for the patient. However, a pressure of 10 cm H_2O was inadequate once REM sleep occurred. A further increase to 12.5 cm H_2O and then 15 cm H_2O was required to reduce the RDI to near normal levels. The patient therefore would have been effectively treated at home if REM sleep or a supine position were present.

As seen in Table 7-2, the patient does not sleep in a supine position until very late in this recording. By the time this occurs, only 45 min sleep remain in the recording and insufficient time is left to properly titrate.

• Patient's subjective response to administration of pressure at a particular level, if available. A patient repeatedly awakened by the sensation of pressure, even if it is objectively successful, may refuse to use this pressure at home. Therefore, a comment that, although the CPAP was objectively successful, the patient tolerated the pressure poorly should be part of the interpretation.

In light of the numerous problems that can be encountered by the patient and sleep technologist in the process of conducting a CPAP titration night, the expectation that sleep disordered breathing will be essentially normalized by CPAP in a single night is quite unrealistic.

TABLE 7-1
Selection of Optimal CPAP Pressure: REM Sleep

	CPAP Pressures (cm H_2O)				
	5	7.5	10	12.5	15.0
RDI	42.5	13.6	4.2	18.0	5.6
REM sleep (min)	20	0	0	36	65

TABLE 7-2
Selection of Optimal CPAP Pressure: Supine Body Position

	CPAP Pressures (cm H_2O)			
	5	7.5	10	12.5
RDI	16.2	6.4	42.7	18.0
Total sleep time (min)	65	346	35	10
Supine sleep (min)	0	0	10	5

TABLE 7-3
Results of CPAP Titration from Figure 7-1

	5 cm H_2O	7.5 cm H_2O	10 cm H_2O	12.5 cm H_2O
Total recording time (min)	19.0	39.5	18.0	387.0*
Total sleep time (min)	9.5	39.5	18.0	358.0
REM sleep (min)	0.0	0.0	2.0	122.5
Total RDI (per hr sleep)	189.5	91.1	36.7	7.0
REM sleep RDI (per hr sleep)	0.0	0.0	90.0	8.3

*Only first 60 min CPAP administration at 12.5 cm H_2O shown in the figure.

Figure 7-1 shows the first 3 hr CPAP titration recording of a 43-year-old man with an overall RDI of 85.5/hr of sleep and a low SaO_2 of <50% during the diagnostic PSG.

Table 7-3 shows the results of CPAP titration on the patient with severe hypoxia studied in Figure 7-1. Administration of the first pressure level of 5 cm H_2O had no effect on the RDI, although, even at this pressure, a low SaO_2 was increased from 75% of the lowest value during NREM sleep on baseline to 84%. A subsequent increase to a pressure of 7.5 cm H_2O resulted in a reduction in the RDI, but it remained well within the range of severe. However, after approximately 30 min of administration at this pressure, the sleep quality began to show improvement. The previously alternating epochs of stage 1 and 2 sleep changed to stage 2 and 3 sleep (see first arrow on left in figure). However, intermittent snoring and hypopneas persisted. An increase to a pressure of 10 cm H_2O resulted in further improvement, but with the onset of REM sleep (middle arrow on figure), significant sleep-disordered breathing returned, with associated O_2 desaturation <90%. For this reason, pressure was increased to 12.5 cm H_2O. As noted in the table, this proved to be successful in limiting the overall RDI and RDI during REM sleep to near normal levels.

SPLIT NIGHT PROTOCOLS

Definition

Split night protocols are a one-night polysomnographic study during which both a diagnostic sleep study and a treatment trial of continuous positive airway pressure are conducted.

General Significance

Split night studies generally are ordered for patients with a strong clinical suspicion of moderate or severe obstructive sleep apnea. Based on the clinical history, the referring physician also makes the a priori decisions that the patient will require treatment and that the best treatment will be CPAP. Split night studies are performed for one of two reasons in the United States:

1. *Logistical.* Sleep disorders center laboratories may have long scheduling delays for sleep studies. Once the patient has been diagnosed with moderate or severe sleep apnea, based on history, a split night study permits confirmation of the diagnosis and treatment without delay.

2. *Financial.* Many health insurance companies or health maintenance organizations (HMO) in the United States attempt to reduce expenditures by limiting access to polysomnography or limiting the number of procedures that can be performed each year.

General Methodology

Split night recording employ identical methodology to both the diagnostic sleep recording and the CPAP treatment trial. They differ only in that often an initial threshold is required for terminating the diagnostic portion of the split night and initiating CPAP administration.

The American Sleep Disorders Association recommends the following protocols:[52]

1. An AHI of at least 40 is documented during a minimum of 2 hr diagnostic polysomnography. Split night studies may be considered at an AHI of 20–40, based on clinical judgment (e.g., if there also are repetitive long obstructions and major desaturation). However, at AHI values below 40, determination of CPAP pressure requirements based on split night studies may be less accurate than in full night calibrations.

2. CPAP titration is carried out for more than 3 hr (because respiratory events can worsen as the night progresses).

3. Polysomnography documents that CPAP eliminates or nearly eliminates the respiratory events during REM and non-REM (NREM) sleep, including REM sleep with the patient in a supine position.

4. A second full night of polysomnography for CPAP titration is performed if the diagnosis of a sleep-related breathing disorder is confirmed but criteria 2 and 3 are not met.

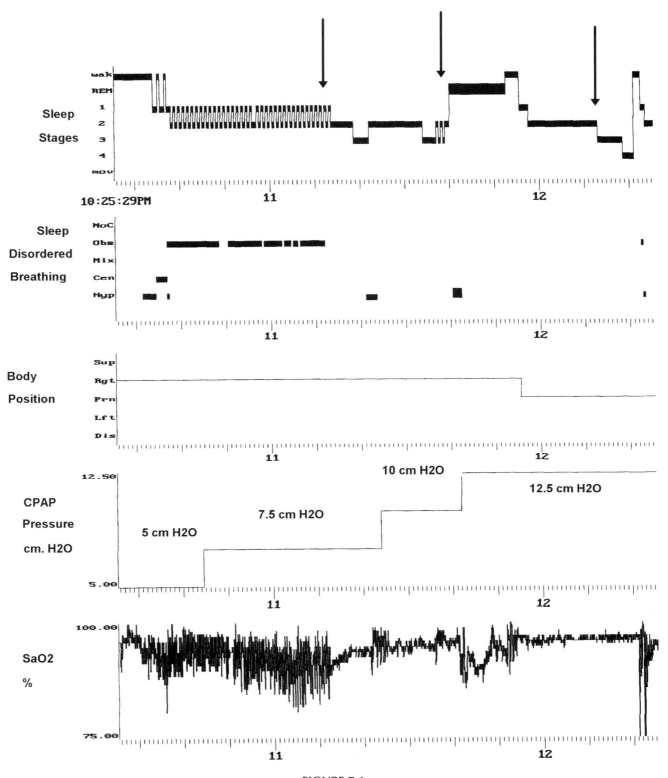

FIGURE 7-1
Typical CPAP titration.

Unfortunately, due to logistical or health insurance based restrictions, only a single night of sleep recording may be available. Although this is the preferred method for conducting split night protocols, alternative protocols with much lower thresholds for initiating CPAP administration may be necessary.

Methodological Concerns

Technically Demanding

Split night studies require the night shift technician to keep a running count of episodes of sleep-disordered breathing and compute the RDI. The technician must awaken the patient in the middle of the sleep period and be prepared to initiate administration of NCPAP, often while simultaneously monitoring other sleep laboratory patients.

Is the Patient Prepared?

Following a full night of diagnostic sleep study, the patient often meets with the physician to discuss the results of the sleep study and to review treatment alternatives. If CPAP is selected as the treatment, the patient receives an orientation and only then is scheduled for a NCPAP treatment trial. With a spilt night recording, the preparation for CPAP treatment may be lacking. If the patient has not been educated about NCPAP, chances increase that CPAP administration will be less successful or fail.

Sufficient Time and Other Concerns

A split night study tries to do in one night what usually would require two nights. It is subject to a much larger range of factors that can contribute to its success or failure. The following factors contribute to success:

- Moderate or severe obstructive sleep apnea present immediately at sleep onset.
- Maximum reduction in sleep-disordered breathing occurs early in the titration process.
- Patient spends sufficient time in bed.
- Patient sleeps a sufficient quantity.
- Patient sleeps in a supine position early in the recording.
- REM sleep is present early in the recording.
- Once the NCPAP mask is positioned and positive pressure started, the patient returns to sleep immediately.
- Patient tolerates the CPAP mask and pressures.
- Patient is not aroused by increased pressure levels during titration.

- Patient is able to breathe nasally.
- Patient does not develop side effects:
  Dry mouth.
  Nasal congestion.
  Facial pain.
  Headache.
  Claustrophobia.
- Technical staff is sufficiently sophisticated, trained, and alert to conduct the protocol and respond to problems as they occur.

These factors contribute to failure:

- Mild sleep apnea.
- NCPAP titration requires administration of numerous pressure levels.
- Optimal reduction in sleep-disordered breathing does not occur due to lack of time.
- Apneas and hypopneas are present primarily during REM sleep or in a supine position.
- REM sleep is absent.
- Patient does not or will not sleep in a supine position.
- No REM sleep present in diagnostic portion of split night.
- No REM sleep present during NCPAP treatment portion of split night.
- No sleep in a supine position during diagnostic portion of split night.
- No sleep in a supine position during NCPAP treatment portion of split night.
- Patient spends insufficient time in bed.
- Patient sleeps an insufficient quantity.
- Once NCPAP mask positioned and positive pressure started, patient is unable to return to sleep.
- Patient is unable to tolerate CPAP mask and pressures.
- Patient is aroused by changes in pressure levels during the titration.
- Patient is unable to breathe nasally.
- Patient develops side effects:
  Dry mouth.
  Nasal congestion.
  Facial pain.
  Headache.
  Claustrophobia.
- Technical staff is not sufficiently sophisticated, trained, and alert to conduct the protocol and respond to problems as they occur.

Figure 7-2 shows histograms of a successful split night recording in a 52-year-old woman. Split night recording was performed as required by her health

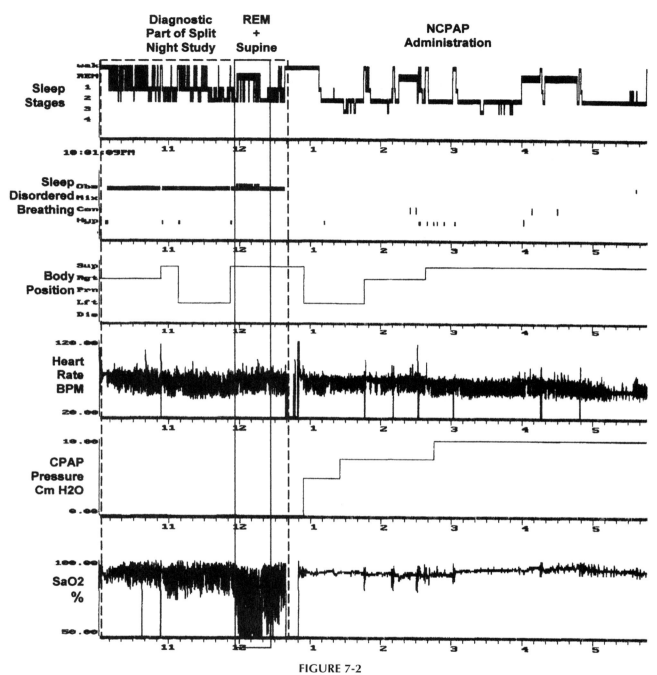

FIGURE 7-2
Successful split night recording.

maintenance organization. This recording has all the features of a successful split night recording:

1. Diagnostic polysomnography was completed in 173 min.
2. Severe sleep apnea was present immediately, with an overall RDI of 96.6/hr of sleep.
3. REM sleep in a supine position occurred approximately 2 hr after sleep onset, allowing for determination of maximum likely severity, including SaO_2 <50%. Patient then could be awakened with the confidence that a diagnosis had been made properly.
4. The CPAP mask was in place early in the recording.
5. The patient returned to sleep <30 min after starting pressure administration.
6. The administration of CPAP was effective immediately, requiring later titration only to eliminate residual snoring and hypopneas during REM sleep.
7. Almost 4 hr relatively uninterrupted sleep present.
8. Patient described her sleep and AM alertness as better than usual.

Case Studies

All the following case studies and case materials are based on actual sleep disorder center cases. However, identifying information has been changed in each case to protect the identity of the patient.

Interpretation of polysomnographic (PSG) data requires not only the raw polysomnographic data and summary statistics but also a variety of other information to properly place the sleep study data in context and determine its reliability and validity. Cases presented here may use one or more of the following:

1. History and physical.
2. Sleep log or diary.
3. Presleep (PM) questionnaire.
4. Postsleep (AM) questionnaire.
5. PSG results or summary data.
6. Multiple Sleep Latency Test data.
7. Technician notes.

Case studies were chosen for three main purposes. The first is for the reader to gain familiarity with the different types of case materials available to the interpreter of sleep studies. The second purpose is for the reader to recognize that polysomnogram interpretation is a *process* that involves evaluating and integrating information from many sources. Third, it is important always to remember that the findings of a diagnostic PSG may or may not be identical to the final diagnosis. The diagnostic polysomnogram plays an important role in ruling out other diagnoses. However, in many cases, the clinical history will be more important than the diagnostic polysomnogram in arriving at the final diagnosis.

The intention of these studies is to suggest *how* the interpreter might arrive at conclusions, not compel any particular conclusion or diagnosis. In reviewing the cases, we suggest the reader imagine a typical fellowship training situation, where a fellow newly introduced to the science and art of polysomnogram interpretation reviews a sleep case along with an experienced sleep specialist who points out items of interest or importance and suggests how they might or might not contribute to reaching a final diagnosis.

Case 1

PRESENTING COMPLAINT

"I fall asleep everywhere."

PATIENT DEMOGRAPHICS

Patient is a 45-year-old, white female, single teacher.

PATIENT SLEEP HISTORY

Onset of excessive daytime sleepiness began during high school, at approximately age 17 years, when she would fall asleep several times a day while seated. Symptoms of sleepiness have worsened over the years, so that she now experiences severe daytime sleepiness throughout the day and may fall asleep any time she is not physically active, even while standing. She currently falls asleep 2–15 times daily, usually for a few seconds with one or two naps exceeding 15 min. She often reports dreams during these naps and finds them refreshing. The 15–30 min following each nap is one of the few times each day she feels relatively alert.

At approximately age 25 years, she began to experience brief periods of muscle weakness following laughter and animated talking. She experiences this as her "knees giving out" followed by a brief dip lasting 1–2 sec. She has never fallen down. She has a similar global sensation on awakening in the morning. She has never experienced this at sleep onset and has never had hallucinations at bedtime or in the morning.

Her family history is positive for an uncle on her father's side known in the family for his "catnapping" and loss of muscle tone with laughing. Her father was known to doze easily, although this appears to have been limited to the evening after dinner.

The patient is unaware of snoring and has not awakened from sleep due to gasping. She breathes nasally and does not awaken with a dry mouth or headache. She experiences no unusual sensations in her lower limbs and is not a fitful sleeper.

SLEEP/WAKE SCHEDULE

During the schoolyear and workweek, the patient reports she gets into bed just before 11 PM and falls to sleep immediately. She typically awakens between 4:30 and 5:30 AM, for a total sleep time of 5.5–6.5 hr. She may awaken once for 5–10 min. On weekends during the schoolyear, she gets into bed at 11 PM and may sleep until 7 or 8 AM for a total sleep time of 8–9 hr. She awakens from sleep during the workweek and weekends feeling alert and refreshed, although these feelings persist for no more than 60 min. The patient believes that the duration of sleep is not related neither to her level of sleepiness during the day nor to the incidence of episodes of muscle weakness.

MEDICAL HISTORY AND EXAM

On exam the patient was 5'5" and 135 lbs. Her weight had changed only 5 lbs in the previous 20 years. Her blood pressure was 135/90 and pulse 70. Neurological, ENT, and mental status exams were unremarkable. She was taking no medication and had taken no prescription medications other than antibiotics for more than 10 years. She expressed a desire to avoid medication for her sleep disorder if at all possible. She had never been hospitalized. On interview, she had no psychological symptoms other than lack of energy.

PRELIMINARY DIAGNOSIS

A history of narcolepsy often does not come any clearer than this one. Directly witnessing a cataplectic attack or the presence of hypnogogic hallucinations are the only additional pieces of data that might further strengthen this history. The chances of this occurring are not high, as only 11% of all patients diagnosed with narcolepsy have all the symptoms in the narcolepsy tetrad.

These are the essential elements of this case consistent with a classic history of narcolepsy:

1. Definite history of excessive daytime sleepiness (EDS) with demand naps starting in the teenage years.
2. Onset of cataplexy 4–5 years after onset of EDS. Cataplexy occurs often enough that the history is not in doubt.
3. Sleep paralysis on awakening.
4. Demand naps are refreshing and associated with dreaming.
5. Positive family history for EDS and possibly cataplexy.
6. Degree of sleepiness is unrelated to the quantity of prior sleep.
7. Nocturnal sleep is refreshing, at least for a short period of time.
8. Patient has no apparent drug-seeking behavior.

Patient had no history suggestive of sleep apnea or periodic leg movements in sleep. However, insufficient sleep may contribute to the patient's complaints. Total sleep times ranging from 5.5–6.5 hr during workweek may result in cumulative partial sleep deprivation.

PLAN

1. Diagnostic polysomnogram (DPSG) to rule out any sleep fragmenting processes, such as sleep apnea or periodic leg movements in sleep.
2. Multiple Sleep Latency Test (MSLT) to objectively confirm patient's complaint of excessive daytime sleepiness and determine if sleep-onset REM periods (SOREMPS) are present.

COMMENTARY ON CLINICAL MATERIALS

All boxed numbers in the figures refer to the comments that follow.

Sleep Log (Figure C1-1)

The sleep log generally confirms the history the patient provided during the initial evaluation. However, the sleep log (Figure C1-1) shows more variability and slightly higher estimated total sleep time. The patient notes that the quality of her sleep was high or moderate, but nevertheless she felt quite fatigued each day. This is most consistent with a sleep disorder not characterized by insufficient sleep.

1. Patient's bedtime occasionally is as early as 9 PM, although she most often goes to bed around 11 PM. Based on this, 11 PM should be the lights out time for the diagnostic polysomnogram.
2. Longer naps are charted and closely resemble the patient's history. However, the 10–15 daily microsleeps or short naps she describes are not charted. This suggests it was just too problematic to chart these brief frequent events and she may not always be aware or remember when they occur.
3. Patient drinks two to three caffeinated beverages, usually between 2:30 and 5 PM and occasionally at other times. This timing may reflect the normal midafternoon "dip." Alternately, this may be a function of her workday. As a middle school teacher, she is actively involved with students and teaching during a schoolday that ends between 2:30 and 3 PM. Therefore, her caffeine use and longer naps on workdays generally occur during a period when she is less physically active.

Bedtime Questionnaire (Figure C1-2)

4. The patient's sleep schedule on the night before diagnostic sleep testing was quite typical of her usual schedule, as noted in her history and on her sleep log. Estimated total sleep time was slightly less than noted on her sleep log but not consistent with any significant sleep deprivation.
5. The patient is confident that she will sleep as well as usual, confirming her history and sleep log data.
6. She followed her typical pattern of caffeine use with three caffeinated beverages between 3:30 and 6 PM. Sudden discontinuation of caffeine could have resulted in withdrawal symptoms.

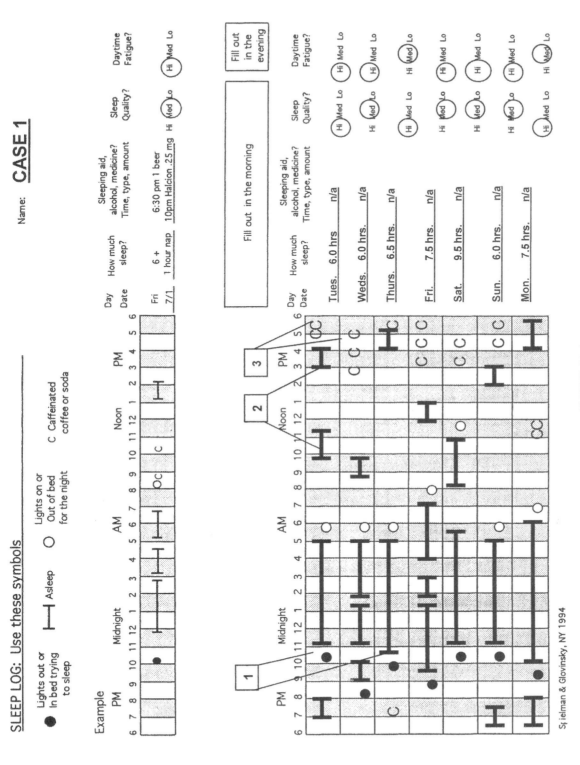

FIGURE C1-1
Sleep log.

BEDTIME QUESTIONNAIRE

How sleepy do you feel right now? Place mark along line.

Very sleepy_____⤬_____ Very Alert

Please describe how you feel now. Circle one of the numbers on the Stanford Sleepiness Scale below:

1. Alert. Wide Awake. Energetic.
2. Functioning at a high level, but not at peak. Able to concentrate.
(3.) Awake, but not fully alert.
4. A little foggy, let down.
5. Foggy. Beginning to lose interest in remaining awake. Slowed down.
6. Cannot stay awake. Sleep onset soon.
7. Asleep

$\boxed{4}$

Please describe your sleep last night:

What time did you turn out the lights?	11:10 PM
How long did it take to fall asleep?	0
How many hours/minutes did you sleep last night?	6
What time did you awaken this morning?	5:10 AM
How many times did you awaken last night?	1

Did you nap or fall asleep today?   (Yes)   No
If YES, please indicate at what times and for how long
About 10 PM for 15 minutes_____

Was today a typical day?   (Yes)   No
If NO, please explain

How well do you expect to sleep tonight? $\boxed{5}$
Same as always – well.

Do you feel ready to go to sleep right now?   (Yes)   No
If NO, please explain

Did you drink any alcohol today?   Yes   (No)

If YES, please list what kind, how much and when taken

Did you drink any caffeinated beverages (coffee, tea, colas, etc.) today? (YES) NO

If YES, please what kind, when taken and how much? $\boxed{6}$
1 coffee at 3:30 PM, cola at 5 PM , tea at 6 PM

FIGURE C1-2
Bedtime (PM) questionnaire, page 1.

Did you smoke any cigarettes, cigars, pipe, etc. today?   YES (NO)

If YES, please what kind, when taken and how much?

_____

Please list all medications you took today. Be sure to include prescriptions medications as well as those you take without a prescription

Name   How Much   Reason   When Taken
None____   _____   _____   _____
_____   _____   _____   _____
_____   _____   _____   _____

Please list any other medication you will be taking before going to sleep

Name   How Much   Reason   When Taken

None   _____   _____   _____
_____   _____   _____   _____
_____   _____   _____   _____

Please list any other medication you have stopped taking in the last 30 days.

Name   How Much   Reason   When Taken

None__   _____   _____   _____
_____   _____   _____   _____
_____   _____   _____   _____

Please describe anything else that occurred last night or today that might affect your sleep tonight. _____Nothing_____
_____

FIGURE C1-2
Bedtime (PM) questionnaire, page 2.

Diagnostic Polysomnogram (Figure C1-3)

7. Lights out time was 12:14 AM, later than was requested and lights on time was 7:02 AM. Therefore, the patient went to bed more than an hour later than usual for her weekend schedule and got out of bed about an hour later than is usual on weekdays or weekends. If the patient's presenting complaint had been difficulty falling asleep or if her complaint suggested a biological rhythm disorder, any delay in the sleep/wake schedule may have resulted in a shortening of sleep latency. This could have influenced the diagnostic importance of the sleep study.

8. Total sleep time was slightly more than 5 hr, fairly typical of the patient's sleep during the workweek but less than on weekends. To rule out insufficient sleep as a significant source of daytime sleepiness, it would have been preferable to have the patient sleep 7+ hr.

9. Stage 1 sleep is within normal limits for a patient of this age during the first night in the sleep laboratory. It certainly does not suggest a repetitive sleep fragmenting process.

10. The total minutes and percentage of deep sleep are higher than expected for a woman of this age during the first night in the sleep laboratory. Its significance is uncertain. Possible explanations include

    Rebound sleep. The sleep log does not document any period of previous partial or acute sleep deprivation or change in sleep/wake schedule other than as already described by the patient.

    Restricted or short sleep pattern. Generally, when sleep is restricted by limiting time in bed to 3–4 hr, deep sleep and REM sleep are preserved at the expense of stage 1 and stage 2 sleep. Therefore, if normal quantities of deep sleep persist during a shorter sleep period, the percentage of deep sleep is likely to increase. This explanation would require that we assume that her 5 hr of total sleep time (TST) or her usual 5.5–6.5 hr is a restricted pattern.

    Normal variant. It may mean nothing. A close examination of normative data at the beginning of this volume shows considerable variation in percentages of deep sleep.

    Unintended treatment effect. A high percentage of deep sleep also may be significant, as it may be associated with a reduced severity of sleep-disordered breathing. It is uncertain if deep sleep suppresses sleep-disordered breathing or deep sleep appears when sleep-disordered breathing ceases.

11. REM sleep latency generally is within normal limits for a patient of this age.

12. Borderline normal obstructive sleep apnea is present, occurring much more frequently during REM sleep.

13. The hypopneas noted were associated with only 3–4% O_2 desaturations with 94% the lowest value noted.

14. Although hypopneas occurred during REM sleep with an index of 14.5/hr, they resulted in minimal disruption of REM sleep. Therefore, it is unlikely that significant REM sleep deprivation has resulted from sleep disordered breathing.

Sample Interpretation

This recording is remarkable for the sleep-disordered breathing. A total of 27 hypopneas were recorded during slightly more than 5 hr of total sleep time for an overall apnea/hypopnea index of 5.3/hr of sleep. Apneas and hypopneas typically were quite short in duration, averaging 17 sec with occasional REM-sleep-related events lasting 37 sec. All events were associated with minimal O_2 desaturation, ranging from 1–4% with 94% the lowest SaO_2 value noted. Occasional soft, rhythmic snoring occurred during REM sleep while in a supine position. EKG was unremarkable. Sleep-disordered breathing was most prominent in association with REM sleep, resulting in a REM sleep index of 14.5/hr.

The overall quality and quantity of sleep was variable. The total sleep time of 5 hr and sleep efficiency of 84% were lower than expected, but deep sleep occurred with a higher percentage than expected. This may reflect rebound sleep or a normal variant.. The patient noted on her morning questionnaire that she had slept worse than usual but had awakened feeling as alert as usual.

In summary, these findings are consistent with mild sleep apnea.

Histograms of Diagnostic Polysomnogram (Figure C1-4)

15. The patient proceeded rapidly into deep sleep and then remained in stage 4 for more than 1 hr. This is not typical of a 45-year-old woman during her first night in the sleep laboratory. The majority of wakefulness also occurred during a single period, starting about around 2:30 AM. Therefore, most

Diagnostic Polysomnogram

7

Lights out: 12:14 AM   Lights on: 7:02 AM

8   **10**   **9**

SLEEP PARAMETERS

GENERAL		
Total Time in Bed	407.5	mins.
Total Sleep Time	**304.0**	mins.
Total Wake Time	103.5	mins.
Sleep Efficiency	**84.0**	%

SLEEP STAGING				
Stage 1	31.0	mins.	10.2	%
Stage 2	98.0	mins.	32.2	%
Stage 3	9.5	mins.	3.1	%
Stage 4	97.0	mins.	32.0	%
REM	68.5	mins.	22.5	%

LATENCIES		
Latency to stage 1	**8.5**	mins.
Latency to stage 2	5.0	mins.
Latency to REM	**84.0**	mins.

WAKETIME		
Wake between sleep onset and sleep offset	93.5	mins.
Wake after sleep offset	1.5	mins.
Awakenings lasting 1-5 mins.	5	
Awakenings > 5 mins.	4	

11

SLEEP DISORDERED BREATHING

	Obstructive		Hypopnea		Central		Totals		
	REM	NREM	REM	NREM	REM	NREM	REM	NREM	All
# of apneas/hypopneas	0	0	16	11	0	0	16	11	27
Index (#/hr. of sleep)			14.5	2.7			14.5	2.7	5.3
Max. Duration (secs)			37	22					
Avg. Duration (secs.)			21	16					
Low SaO2 (%)			94	95					
Avg. SaO2 (%)			97	97					
Avg. Arousal (secs.)			4	18					

12   **13**

14 BASELINE CARDIORESPIRATORY DATA

	Wake		REM		NREM	
ECG	58-105		60-80		50-72	
Respiratory Rate	13-15		15-18		15-17	
SaO2*	97-100	%	96-97	%**	95-98	%

FIGURE C1-3
Polysomnogram (DPSG) report, page 1.

OTHER CARDIORESPIRATORY DATA

Body Position: Sleep was recorded while in the right and left lateral decubitus and supine positions.

Post Apnea/hypopnea arousals: Usually ranged 3-45 seconds.

Undisturbed sleep: Approximately 4.0 hours while in all positions during NREM sleep.

Snoring: There was soft, rhythmic snoring during REM sleep while supine.

Arrhythmias: None.

MOVEMENT PARAMETERS

	#	Index	
Total periodic leg movements in sleep (PLMS)	0	0	per hour of sleep
PLMS resulting in arousal			per hour of sleep
Duration of arousals	-	seconds	
Total nonperiodic leg movements in sleep (NPLMS)	0	0	per hour of sleep
NPLMS resulting in arousal			per hour of sleep
Duration of arousals	-	seconds	

ADDITIONAL FINDINGS

The patient reported sleeping worse than usual.

MEDICATIONS

Type	Amount	When taken
None		

FIGURE C1-3
Polysomnogram (DPSG) report, page 2.

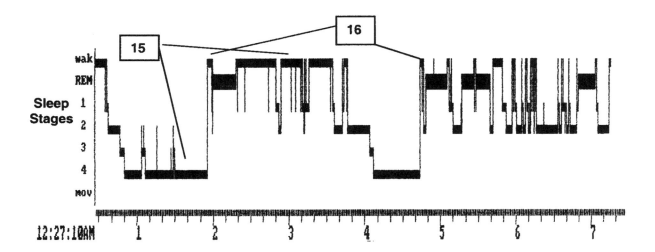

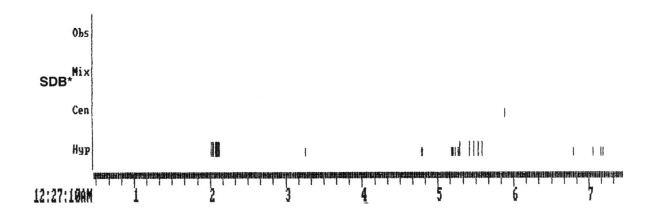

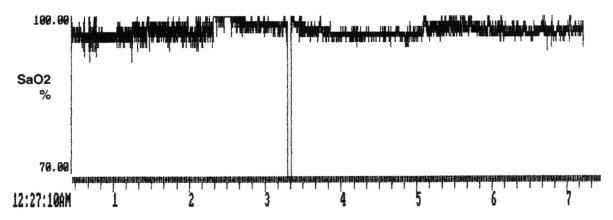

FIGURE C1-4
Polysomnogram (DPSG) histogram.

wakefulness is not due to frequent, brief arousals, as might result from sleep apnea or periodic leg movements in sleep.

16. The patient was awakened twice from stage 4 sleep by hypopneas and within 5 min entered REM sleep. In the classical description of sleep stage cycling, REM sleep follows a period of stage 2 sleep. It has been occasionally noted that patients with narcolepsy frequently enter REM sleep following some disruption to sleep or directly following wakefulness or stage 1 sleep.

Morning Questionnaire (Figure C1-5)

17. The patient reported sleeping worse than usual. This is a probable first night effect (FNE) and reflects the difficulty of sleeping in a laboratory setting for the first time. However, the patient also reported awakening with her usual level of alertness. These answers may not seem consistent at first, but the second question allows the patient to focus on how he or she is feeling at that moment, while the first requires the patient to take into consideration the entire experience of sleeping in a sleep laboratory, including the sensors, bed, noise, and so forth.

18. This confirms the objective findings of the DPSG and the differences from the patient's usual sleep at home.

Multiple Sleep Latency Test (Figure C1-6)

19. A mean sleep latency of 7.3 min is consistent with moderately severe daytime sleepiness but is longer than reported for most patients with narcolepsy.

20. The sleep latency at the 2 PM nap may have been influenced by the activities surrounding a later-than-planned lunch. Walking up and back to the laboratory kitchenette may have activated her and resulted in an increased sleep latency.

21. Unambiguous REM sleep was noted shortly after sleep onset in each of the four naps. In the absence of any other significant sleep disorder or explanation for the appearance of these sleep-onset REM periods (SOREMPs), they are strong evidence for a diagnosis of narcolepsy.

Sample Interpretation

A mean sleep latency of 7.3 min (to stage 1 sleep) is consistent with the finding of moderate daytime sleepiness but slightly longer than usually found in patients with narcolepsy. However, the presence of REM sleep in all four naps is most consistent with the diagnosis of narcolepsy.

MORNING QUESTIONNAIRE

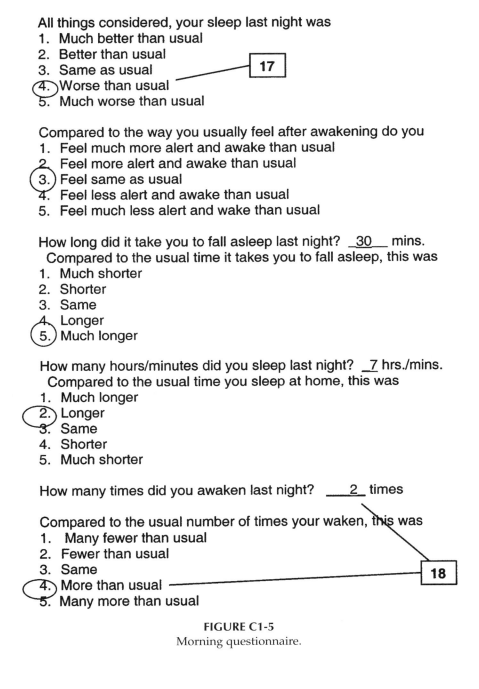

All things considered, your sleep last night was
1. Much better than usual
2. Better than usual
3. Same as usual   17
4. Worse than usual
5. Much worse than usual

Compared to the way you usually feel after awakening do you
1. Feel much more alert and awake than usual
2. Feel more alert and awake than usual
3. Feel same as usual
4. Feel less alert and awake than usual
5. Feel much less alert and wake than usual

How long did it take you to fall asleep last night? __30__ mins.
  Compared to the usual time it takes you to fall asleep, this was
1. Much shorter
2. Shorter
3. Same
4. Longer
5. Much longer

How many hours/minutes did you sleep last night? _7_ hrs./mins.
  Compared to the usual time you sleep at home, this was
1. Much longer
2. Longer
3. Same
4. Shorter
5. Much shorter

How many times did you awaken last night? ___2_ times

Compared to the usual number of times your waken, this was
1. Many fewer than usual
2. Fewer than usual
3. Same
4. More than usual   18
5. Many more than usual

FIGURE C1-5
Morning questionnaire.

MULTIPLE SLEEP LATENCY TEST (MSLT) REPORT

TEST RESULTS

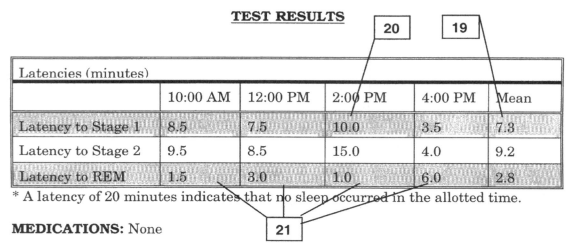

Latencies (minutes)					
	10:00 AM	12:00 PM	2:00 PM	4:00 PM	Mean
Latency to Stage 1	8.5	7.5	10.0	3.5	7.3
Latency to Stage 2	9.5	8.5	15.0	4.0	9.2
Latency to REM	1.5	3.0	1.0	6.0	2.8

* A latency of 20 minutes indicates that no sleep occurred in the allotted time.

MEDICATIONS: None

ADDITIONAL DATA: The patient reported that she was as alert as usual during the test. The patient had lunch at 1:00 PM.

FIGURE C1-6
MSLT report page.

FINAL SYNTHESIS

The patient's history of excessive daytime sleepiness and cataplexy were powerful clinical evidence for the diagnosis of narcolepsy. Although the diagnostic polysomnogram raised some issues that required working through, it ruled out other significant sleep disorders that could have been the sole source of the patient's daytime sleepiness or contributed to it. It also laid the groundwork for interpreting the MSLT.

It should be remembered that sleep disorders noted during diagnostic sleep studies are not always consistent with the final diagnoses. In this case, the diagnostic polysomnogram ruled out other sleep disorders, although it did raise the possibility of prior sleep deprivation.

On the basis of these findings, along with the strong clinical history for narcolepsy, the sleep disorders center staff felt secure in the final diagnosis of narcolepsy.

Case 2

PRESENTING COMPLAINT

"I am tired all day long, every day."

PATIENT DEMOGRAPHICS

Patient is a single, 26-year-old African-American female working as a dental assistant.

PATIENT SLEEP HISTORY

The patient states she has been sleepy as long as she can remember. She was noted for dozing frequently during classes, especially if bored. The patient also may doze while at work, while watching TV or movies, and while reading. The patient does not report dozing while driving.

The patient takes one or two planned naps per day, each lasting 20–40 min. Additionally, she may fall asleep briefly two or three times daily. All naps generally are refreshing, and she reports that vivid dreaming occurs during both planned and unplanned naps.

The patient reports loss of muscle tone in her legs and arms following laughter, occurring primarily in the last two to three years. These occur several times a week and occasionally result in a fall to the floor. The patient denies experiencing sleep paralysis or hypnogogic hallucinations.

Neither parent has similar symptoms, although a sister was diagnosed with "chronic fatigue syndrome" at another hospital.

The patient is unaware of snoring and has not awakened gasping or choking. However, she experiences chronic nasal congestion and has awakened with a dry mouth since childhood.

SLEEP/WAKE SCHEDULE

The patient reports sleeping 7–8 hr during the workweek and as many as 10 hr on days off. Despite the increased sleep on weekends, she generally awakens feeling alert and functioning at a high level, although not at her peak on both weekdays and weekends. Within an hour, she feels quite sleepy no matter what the duration of the prior night's sleep. The patient reports no awakenings from sleep most nights.

MEDICAL HISTORY AND EXAM

On exam, the patient was 5'4" and 122 lbs. Her blood pressure was 122/81 and pulse 71 and regular. Her ENT examination and neurological examination were unremarkable. She was taking no medication and had never taken prescription medication other than antibiotics. She had never been hospitalized. On interview, she had no signs or symptoms of depression or other psychological disorder. She appeared very interested in the proper diagnosis of her disorder but stated she was not willing to take medication of any sort for her problem.

PRELIMINARY DIAGNOSES

- *Narcolepsy.* The patients presenting symptoms appear highly consistent with the diagnosis of narcolepsy. She has a long history of excessive daytime sleepiness, associated only in the last 2–3 years with the onset of clear cataplexy. This is consistent, as cataplexy most often appears several years after the onset of daytime sleepiness. Other auxiliary symptoms are not present, but they are less significant than cataplexy and daytime sleepiness.

- *Insufficient sleep or a long sleeper.* The patient reports a significant increase in her time in bed and total sleep time on days off. This pattern often is noted in patients who restrict their sleep and time in bed during the workweek only to increase sleep time on days off. However, the patient reports sleeping 7–8 hr during the workweek. If this is insufficient for her needs, she may be a long sleeper, in need of 9–10 hr of sleep.
- *Obstructive sleep apnea.* As a young, thin, premenopausal woman, the patient is at very low risk for sleep apnea. She additionally has none of the usual signs and symptoms: snore-related arousals, gasping, AM headache. However, she has experienced significant nasal congestion, resulting in oral breathing with a dry mouth every morning.

PLAN

To provide objective support for the diagnosis of narcolepsy and rule out the possible presence of obstructive sleep apnea through

1. Diagnostic polysomnogram (DPSG).
2. Multiple Sleep Latency Test (MSLT).

COMMENTARY ON CLINICAL MATERIALS

All boxed numbers in the figures refer to the comments that follow.

Sleep Log (Figure C2-1)

1. The sleep log documents longer duration sleep than she reported in her initial evaluation. Workweek nights she estimated her total sleep time as 8.2–9.5 hr. On weekend nights, she estimated her total sleep time between 9.5 and 10.5 hr.
2. The patient noted one to three naps, lasting 30–70 min each. Most of these occurred between 2–4 PM and 6–8 PM. She did not note any of the shorter "microsleeps" she described on interview. During the 2–4 PM period, caffeine use also was common.
3. The patient describes her sleep as high in quality and did not insert even a single period of wakeful-

ness on her log. Despite the high quality of sleep, she described her level of daytime fatigue as medium or high on five of the seven days charted. The fatigue ratings do not appear related to either the quantity or quality of sleep.

Bedtime Questionnaire (Figure C2-2)

4. The patient decided, without informing sleep laboratory personnel, to take a vacation week during which her testing would take place. She started her vacation two days prior to testing and kept a "weekend" schedule before testing awakening at 10:00 AM after 9 hr continuous sleep. If the patient had established this as her regular schedule, it would require a shift in the timing of her planned DPSG and MSLT to later times. Starting the MSLT at 10:00 AM would have meant putting the patient to sleep at the time she ordinarily would be awakening. As REM sleep occurs in greater quantities toward the end of the usual sleep period, the chances for a SOREMP during the 10:00 AM nap would be significantly increased.
5. The patient reported no napping, despite reporting the day as "typical." This is unusual, as at least one long nap is charted on each of the seven days of the sleep log. Its significance is uncertain.

Diagnostic Polysomnogram (Figure C2-3)

6. Lights out and lights on times are consistent with her usual weekday times. The sudden change in lights out from 1 AM the night before to 11:25 PM on the night of the study could have resulted in a long sleep latency if the patient had phase delayed to 1 AM time as her biological bedtime. The fact that she fell asleep in 16 min argues against this.
7. A total sleep time of 6.7 hr was noted. This is at least 1.5 hr less than any of the total sleep times the patient noted on her sleep log but close to the 7–8 hr of sleep reported in her initial evaluation. The possibility of a 15–20% reduction in total sleep time for one night should be kept in mind in interpreting the sleep latencies on the MSLT.
8. The quality of sleep generally is within normal limits for a 26-year-old woman during her first night in a sleep laboratory.
9. REM sleep latency is statistically shorter than expected but of uncertain clinical significance. It is longer than usually reported for narcolepsy or a major affective disorder. However, smaller changes in REM sleep latency can occur following changes

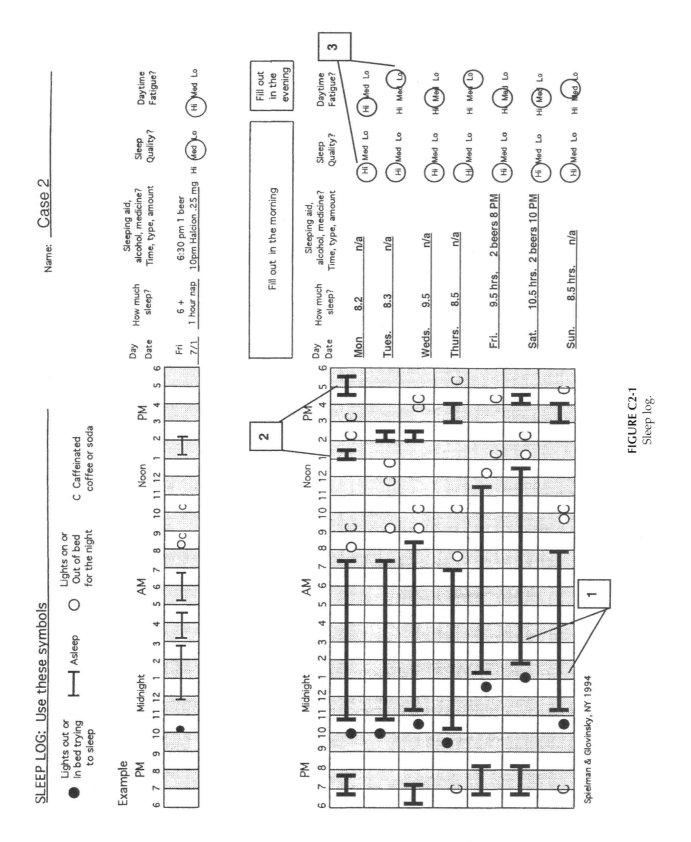

FIGURE C2-1
Sleep log.

BEDTIME QUESTIONNAIRE

How sleepy do you feel right now? Place mark along line.

Very sleepy_____ Very Alert

Please describe how you feel now. Circle one of the numbers on the Stanford Sleepiness Scale below:

1. Alert. Wide Awake. Energetic.
2. Functioning at a high level, but not at peak. Able to concentrate.
3. Awake, but not fully alert.
4. A little foggy, let down.
5. Foggy. Beginning to lose interest in remaining awake. Slowed down.
6. Cannot stay awake. Sleep onset soon.

Please describe your sleep last night:

What time did you turn out the lights?	1:00 AM
How long did it take to fall asleep?	2 mins.
How many hours/minutes did you sleep last night?	9 hrs.
What time did you awaken this morning?	10:00 AM
How many times did you awaken last night?	0

4

Did you nap or fall asleep today?   Yes   No
If YES, please indicate at what times and for how long

5

Was today a typical day?   Yes   No
If NO, please explain

How well do you expect to sleep tonight?
Well

Do you feel ready to go to sleep right now?   Yes   No
If NO, please explain

Did you drink any alcohol today?   Yes   No
If YES, please list what kind, how much and when taken

Did you drink any caffeinated beverages (coffee, tea, colas, etc.) today? YES NO
If YES, please what kind, when taken and how much?
2 coffees 10 AM and 3 PM

FIGURE C2-2
Bedtime questionnaire, page 1.

Did you smoke any cigarettes, cigars, pipe, etc. today?   YES NO

Please list all medications you took today. Be sure to include prescriptions medications as well as those you take without a prescription

Name	How Much	Reason	When Taken
None			

Please list any other medication you will be taking before going to sleep

Name	How Much	Reason	When Taken
None			

Please list any other medication you have stopped taking in the last 30 days.

Name	How Much	Reason	When Taken
None			

Please describe anything else that occurred last night or today that might affect your sleep tonight. ___Nothing___

FIGURE C2-2
Bedtime questionnaire, page 2.

Diagnostic Polysomnogram

Lights out: 11:25 PM   Lights on: 6: 51 AM

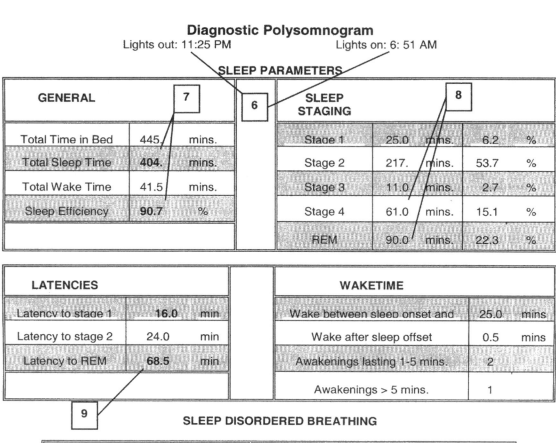

SLEEP PARAMETERS

GENERAL			7	6	SLEEP STAGING				8
Total Time in Bed	445.	mins.			Stage 1	25.0	mins.	6.2	%
Total Sleep Time	**404.**	mins.			Stage 2	217.	mins.	53.7	%
Total Wake Time	41.5	mins.			Stage 3	11.0	mins.	2.7	%
Sleep Efficiency	**90.7**	%			Stage 4	61.0	mins.	15.1	%
					REM	90.0	mins.	22.3	%

LATENCIES				WAKETIME		
Latency to stage 1	**16.0**	min		Wake between sleep onset and	25.0	mins
Latency to stage 2	24.0	min		Wake after sleep offset	0.5	mins
Latency to REM	**68.5**	min		Awakenings lasting 1-5 mins.	2	
				Awakenings > 5 mins.	1	

9

SLEEP DISORDERED BREATHING

	Obstructive		Hypopnea		Central		Totals		
	REM	NREM	REM	NREM	REM	NREM	REM	NREM	All
# of apneas/hypopneas	0	0	14	2	3	3	17	5	22
Index (#/hr. of sleep)			9.3	0.3	2.0	0.5	11.3	1.0	3.3
Max. Duration (secs)			25	27	21	18			
Avg. Duration (secs.)			16	21	18	14			
Low SaO2 (%)			95	97	96	97			
Avg. SaO2 (%)			97	97	97	98			
Avg. Arousal (secs.)			5	25	8	10			

10

11

BASELINE CARDIORESPIRATORY DATA

	Wake	REM	NREM
ECG	48-73	54-70	45-59
Respiratory Rate	14-19	14-20	14-15
SaO2*	99-100 %	98-99 %	97-100 %

FIGURE C2-3
Polysomnogram (DPSG) report, page 1.

OTHER CARDIORESPIRATORY DATA

Body Position: The patient slept in the supine and, right and left lateral decubitus positions.

Undisturbed sleep: Approximately 5 hours.

Snoring: Only soft snoring was noted. ──────────────── 12

Arrhythmias: Rare PVCs.

MOVEMENT PARAMETERS

	#	Index	
Total periodic leg movements in sleep (PLMS)	0	0	per hour of sleep
PLMS resulting in arousal			per hour of sleep
Duration of arousals		seconds	
Total nonperiodic leg movements in sleep (NPLMS)	0	0	per hour of sleep
NPLMS resulting in arousal			per hour of sleep
Duration of arousals		seconds	

ADDITIONAL FINDINGS

The patient reported sleeping worse than usual, but awakened feeling more alert than usual.

MEDICATIONS

Type	Amount	When taken
Vitamin C		

FIGURE C2-3
Polysomnogram (DPSG) report, page 2.

in sleep/wake schedule and withdrawal from REM-sleep-suppressing medications. REM sleep rebound following discontinuation of REM-sleep-suppressing medication is maximum for 2–3 days but can continue above baseline levels for weeks.

10. Sleep-disordered breathing is present but does not meet the usual 5/hr threshold for the diagnosis of obstructive sleep apnea. However, the majority of hypopneas and central apneas noted occur during REM sleep, causing minor REM sleep fragmentation.

11. There is no strict rule for assessing the impact of arousals on REM sleep, but 17 arousals lasting 5 sec each during 90 min REM sleep would appear to be insufficient to cause significant REM sleep deprivation. Additionally, hypopneas and central apneas were associated with minimal O_2 desaturation of 3–4%.

12. Snoring was noted but soft.

Sample Interpretation

This recording was generally within normal limits for a patient of this age. Sleep-disordered breathing was present but did not meet the threshold for the diagnosis of obstructive sleep apnea. A total of 22 apneas and hypopneas were recorded for an overall respiratory disturbance index of 3.3/hr of sleep. Apneas and hypopneas averaged 15 sec in duration, with occasional apneas and hypopneas persisting for 27 sec. Apneas and hypopneas were associated with 3–4% O_2 desaturations with 95% the lowest SaO_2 value noted. Very soft snoring was noted intermittently. ECG was remarkable for rare PVCs.

The quality of sleep was within normal limits for a patient of this age. Light stage 1 sleep accounted for less than 7% of total sleep time. Deep sleep and rapid eye movement (REM) sleep generally were within normal limits for the first night in a sleep laboratory. Brief arousals from sleep occurred following each of the apneas and hypopneas but did not result in significant fragmentation of sleep. The patient reported sleeping worse than usual but awakened feeling more alert than usual. REM sleep typically occurs 90–120 min after sleep onset. A REM sleep latency of 68.5 min, as noted in this recording, is shorter than expected. REM sleep latencies in this range could be associated with affective disorders, circadian rhythm disorders, recent discontinuation

of REM-sleep-suppressing medication, recent elimination of REM-sleep-fragmenting processes or relief of recent acute or cumulative partial sleep deprivation.

In summary, the quality and quantity of sleep were within normal limits for a patient of this age.

Histogram (Figure C2-4)

13. The overall architecture of sleep appears normal for the first night in a sleep laboratory. REM sleep appears for the first time 68.5 min after sleep onset and follows a normal but short non-REM (NREM) cycle. REM sleep during this first REM period is disrupted by an arousal secondary to a hypopnea.

14. Hypopneas and central apneas are concentrated during periods of REM sleep. Using the stacked histograms this easily can be seen by following periods of REM sleep downward.

15. SaO_2 artifacts occur during a period with several awakenings. This type of sudden O_2 desaturation might be possible during REM sleep but certainly not during wakefulness.

Morning Questionnaire (Figure C2-5)

16. The patient reports that, all things considered, she slept worse than usual but awakened feeling more alert than usual. This may appear inconsistent, as the patient could find little about the sleep laboratory environment that was the same as at home. The two questions are considerably different. The second one forces the patient to focus on one particular moment and make a statement about her alertness at that moment. This statement could reflect improved quantity or quality of the prior night's sleep compared to her usual sleep. However, her prior sleep, as noted in her sleep log, would appear to be longer and better in quality. Therefore, her statement might reflect the effect laboratory procedures had on her alertness immediately after awakening. On awakening in her home environment, it is unlikely that someone asks her to fill in questionnaires or removes electrodes and sensors.

17. The patient overestimated her total sleep time as 8 hr compared to the 6.7 hr objectively recorded. If this is a common feature of her subjective estimations of sleep, then her sleep log may be an overestimation of time spent actually sleeping. As noted in comment 3, the patient charted no periods of wakefulness during sleep.

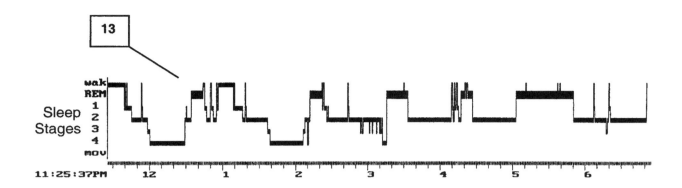

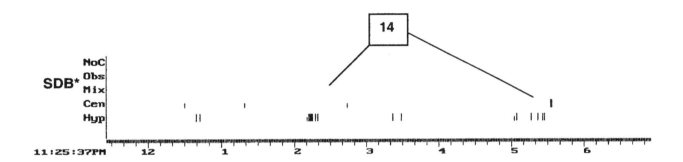

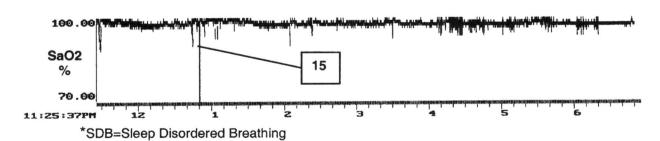

*SDB=Sleep Disordered Breathing

FIGURE C2-4
DPSG histogram.

MORNING QUESTIONNAIRE

All things considered, your sleep last night was

(circle one answer)

1. Much better than usual
2. Better than usual
3. Same as usual
4. Worse than usual
5. Much worse than usual ――― 16

Compared to the way you usually feel after awakening do you

1. Feel much more alert and awake than usual
2. Feel more alert and awake than usual
3. Feel same as usual
4. Feel less alert and awake than usual
5. Feel much less alert and wake than usual

How long did it take you to fall asleep last night? 15-20 mins.

Compared to the usual time it takes you to fall asleep, this was
1. Much shorter
2. Shorter
3. Same
4. Longer
5. Much longer

How many hours/minutes did you sleep last night? 8.0 hrs./mins.

Compared to the usual time you sleep at home, this was
1. Much longer
2. Longer
3. Same ――――――――― 17
4. Shorter
5. Much shorter

How many times did you awaken last night? 4 times

Compared to the usual number of times your waken, this was
1. Many fewer than usual
2. Fewer than usual
3. Same
4. More than usual 18
5. Many more than usual

FIGURE C2-5
Morning questionnaire, page 1.

Please comment specifically on how your night in the sleep laboratory was different from sleep at home

	Circle one	Describe
Room Temperature	Better Same (Worse)	_____
Mattress	Better Same (Worse)	_____
Pillow	Better Same (Worse)	_____
Noise	Better Same (Worse)	_____
Light	Better Same (Worse)	_____
Sleeping Position	Better Same (Worse)	_____
Blankets	Better Same (Worse)	_____
Sense of Security	Better Same (Worse)	_____
Snacks	Better Same (Worse)	_____
TV	Better (Same) Worse	_____
_____	Better Same Worse	_____
_____	Better Same Worse	_____

In what way was your sleep or the sleeping environment better here than your bedroom at home? _____n/a_____

In what way was your sleep or the sleeping environment worse here than your bedroom at home? Awakened many more times than usual, nose was not congested.   19

Did anything happen in the sleep laboratory (other than electrodes etc.) that does not usually happen at home? Bed was too small_____

Does anything usually happen at home during sleep that did not happen here? ___Electrodes_____

How was the sleep test different from what you expected? _Was as expected.

Any comments or suggestions? _____

FIGURE C2-5
Morning questionnaire, page 2.

18. Paradoxically, the patient did report four awakenings during the sleep recording, making speculation about her apparent misperception or lack of memory regarding wakefulness during sleep difficult to support.

19. Although she awakened many more times than usual, these awakenings largely were unrelated to sleep-disordered breathing. This may be due to the lack of nasal congestion during this recording, which could have reduced the severity of sleep-disordered breathing. However, a REM sleep hypopnea did result in the arousal that preceded the major period of wakefulness in this recording (see comment 13).

Multiple Sleep Latency Test (Figure C2-6)

20. A mean sleep latency of 10.3 min is at the usual threshold between moderate and mild sleepiness. It would be atypical for a patient with narcolepsy.

21. The patient failed to fall asleep on the last nap. This is not an unusual phenomenon, even for patients who appear to be severely sleepy during the preceding naps. Generally, it appears to result from the patient's anticipation or anxiety about leaving the laboratory after 20+ hr and regarding the results. In our laboratory, we call this phenomenon the *cabin fever effect*. Generally, when the patient is unable to fall asleep on the last nap and this is considerably different from sleep latencies in preceding naps, strong consideration should be given to excluding it from computation of the mean. With exclusion of the last sleep latency, the mean would be 7.9 min. This is in the range of moderate daytime sleepiness but still longer than reported for patients with narcolepsy. Repetition of the DPSG and MSLT might be indicated, as previous studies have reported that MSLT results may vary from day to day. The numbers of sleep-onset REM periods (SOREMPs) also may increase or decrease.

22. A single sleep-onset REM period occurred during the fourth nap. A single SOREMP is not considered consistent with a diagnosis of narcolepsy. Single SOREMPs have been reported in a wide variety of normal clinical sleep studies. For this reason, at least two SOREMPs usually are required to support a diagnosis of narcolepsy. However, this rule has come into debate following the recent publication of data that showed some normal controls can have as many as two SOREMPs.[86] Despite this, the presence of a single SOREMP in nap 4 is much less common in my experience than a single SOREMP in nap 1 or 2.

Sample Interpretation

A mean sleep latency of 10.3 min (to stage 1 sleep) is consistent with a finding of borderline normal alertness. The patient failed to fall asleep on the fifth nap, a not uncommon finding. If this nap is excluded, the mean sleep latency is 7.9 min, consistent with moderate daytime sleepiness. The presence of REM sleep in one of five of the naps has been reported in normal controls and patients with other sleep disorders. Therefore, these findings do not support a diagnosis of narcolepsy, but cannot rule it out.

MULTIPLE SLEEP LATENCY TEST (MSLT) REPORT

DESCRIPTION OF PROCEDURES: The MSLT consists of 5 twenty minute nap opportunities given at 2 hour intervals throughout the course of one day. Patients are instructed to fall asleep as quickly as possible. If sleep occurs the nap is terminated 15 minutes after sleep onset. Patients are not permitted to sleep between scheduled naps. All data are visually scored and analyzed according to standard criteria.

TEST RESULTS

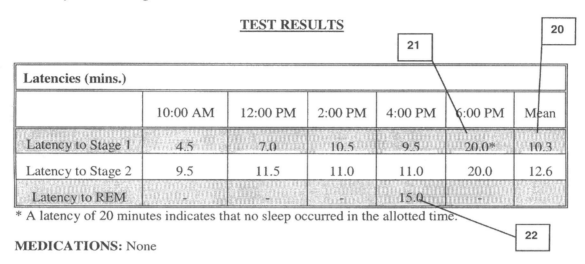

Latencies (mins.)						
	10:00 AM	12:00 PM	2:00 PM	4:00 PM	6:00 PM	Mean
Latency to Stage 1	4.5	7.0	10.5	9.5	20.0*	10.3
Latency to Stage 2	9.5	11.5	11.0	11.0	20.0	12.6
Latency to REM	-	-	-	15.0	-	

* A latency of 20 minutes indicates that no sleep occurred in the allotted time.

MEDICATIONS: None

ADDITIONAL DATA: The patient reported that she was as alert as usual during the day.

FIGURE C2-6
MSLT report.

FINAL SYNTHESIS

The patient's history is highly consistent with the diagnosis of narcolepsy. The presence of cataplexy is definitive. The patient exhibits no drug-seeking behavior or previous history of drug abuse that would lead one to believe that this history was provided as a means of securing a prescription for amphetamines or similar drugs. The sleep log suggests that the patient is sleeping 8–10 high-quality hours each night. This should rule out insufficient sleep as a cause of her sleepiness. The DPSG rules out the most other common sleep disorders, such as sleep apnea or periodic leg movements in sleep. The MSLT provides the least support for the diagnosis of narcolepsy. Even with the fifth nap eliminated, the mean sleep latency is longer than expected and only a single SOREMP was present. Although the MSLT is an important part of the diagnostic workup, a clear history of cataplexy is clinically more important. In this case, the MSLT would have been confirmatory. In cases in which the patient presents with sleepiness of unknown origin without cataplexy, the MSLT would play a more central role.

Of course, the physician who potentially will be prescribing analeptic medications to this patient certainly may prefer some objective confirmation of the diagnosis. Repeat diagnostic testing might produce the desired confirmation of severe daytime sleepiness and more than two SOREMPs, or it might not. If the prescribing physician does not feel strongly about this objective confirmation, then the diagnosis of narcolepsy should be made with the available strong clinical data.

Case 3

PRESENTING COMPLAINT

"I am falling asleep while driving."

Patient was referred by HMO physician unaffiliated with Sleep Disorders Center with request to perform diagnostic polysomnography followed by a MSLT to rule out narcolepsy. The physician refused to send patient for consultation with Sleep Disorders Center staff. He provided the following information.

PATIENT DEMOGRAPHICS

The patient is a 31-year-old male, a teacher who commutes to work by car each day, 1.5 hr in each direction.

PATIENT SLEEP HISTORY

The patient has experienced excessive daytime sleepiness since at least age 18 years.

SLEEP/WAKE SCHEDULE

Unknown, sleep log not filled out.

MEDICAL HISTORY AND EXAM

The patient is 5'6" and 165 lbs. Neurological and mental status exams reported as normal. There is no past history of drug abuse. Current medication is Prozac only, recently prescribed for "depression" following a divorce. No other medical history provided.

PLAN

As ordered by the referring physician,

1. Diagnostic polysomnogram (DPSG).
2. Multiple Sleep Latency Test (MSLT).

COMMENTARY ON CLINICAL MATERIALS

All numbers on the figures refer to the comments that follow.

Sleep Log

No sleep log was provided by the patient or referring physician. Therefore, the only data available are on the patient's sleep the night before coming to the sleep laboratory. This is presented in the Bedtime Questionnaire. Hence, it is difficult to rule out insufficient sleep or a biological rhythm disorder.

Bedtime Questionnaire (Figure C3-1)

1. The bedtime questionnaire typically is given to the patient 30 min prior to bedtime. At 10:45 PM, the patient rated himself at number 6, the sleepiest rating, on the Stanford Sleep Scale (SSS).
2. The Bedtime Questionnaire indicates that the patient estimates he slept 6 hr the night before sleep testing and took 45 min to fall asleep. This long

113

BEDTIME QUESTIONNAIRE

How sleepy do you feel right now? Place mark along line.

Very sleepy ✕——————————————— Very Alert

Please describe how you feel now. Circle one of the numbers on the Stanford Sleepiness Scale below:

1. Alert. Wide Awake. Energetic.
2. Functioning at a high level, but not at peak. Able to concentrate.
3. Awake, but not fully alert.
4. A little foggy, let down.
5. Foggy. Beginning to lose interest in remaining awake. Slowed down.
6. Cannot stay awake. Sleep onset soon.

Please describe your sleep last night:

| | | **1** |

What time did you turn out the lights?   12:30 AM
How long did it take to fall asleep?   45 mins.
How many hours/minutes did you sleep last night?   6.0
What time did you awaken this morning?   6:30 AM
How many times did you awaken last night?   4

Did you nap or fall asleep today?   Yes   No
If YES, please indicate at what times and for how long
    15 mins X 2

Was today a typical day?   Yes   No
If NO, please explain

How well do you expect to sleep tonight?
Good

Do you feel ready to go to sleep right now?   Yes   No
If NO, please explain

Did you drink any alcohol today?   Yes   No

If YES, please list what kind, how much and when taken

Did you drink any caffeinated beverages (coffee, tea, colas, etc.) today? YES NO
If YES, please what kind, when taken and how much?

FIGURE C3-1
Bedtime questionnaire, page 1.

Did you smoke any cigarettes, cigars, pipe, etc. today?   YES (NO)

5 | If YES, please what kind, when taken and how much?

_____

Please list all medications you took today. Be sure to include prescriptions medications as well as those you take without a prescription

Name	How Much	Reason	When Taken
Dexedrine	5 mg x 6	sleepiness	8-11:30 AM
Birthcontrol			

Please list any other medication you will be taking before going to sleep

Name	How Much	Reason	When Taken
None			

6 | Please list any other medication you have stopped taking in the last 30 days.

Name	How Much	Reason	When Taken
Dexedrine Spansule 15 mg. x 2		sleepiness	

Please describe anything else that occurred last night or today that might affect your sleep tonight. _____ None _____

_____

FIGURE C3-1
Bedtime questionnaire, page 2.

sleep latency appears unusual in someone presenting with severe excessive daytime sleepiness.

3. The patient notes awakening four times during the prior night's sleep, suggesting some sleep fragmenting process, such as sleep apnea.

4. The patient reported two naps, although the timing and duration of these naps was omitted.

5. The patient noted on his questionnaire that he had taken 30 mg dexedrine on the morning of the sleep study. This is highly significant, in that the referring physician apparently failed to supervise the discontinuation of this medication and failed to inform the sleep laboratory. Dexedrine is of special concern, in that it is both an alerting and REM-sleep-suppressing medication and could affect both the diagnostic polysomnogram and the MSLT scheduled the next day. When dexedrine is discontinued suddenly, a REM sleep rebound can occur that would make interpretation of the diagnostic polysomnogram and MSLT difficult or impossible.

6. The patient further notes that he had discontinued an additional 30 mg dexedrine given as 15 mg spansules. Therefore, the patient may have taken 60 mg dexedrine up to the day before the sleep study. At best, the patient had suddenly reduced his dose of dexedrine from 60 mg to 30 mg.

Diagnostic Polysomnogram (Figure C3-2)

7. The quantity and percentage of stage 1 sleep is well within the normal range, suggesting that a sleep fragmenting process, such as sleep apnea or periodic leg movements in sleep, is not present.

8. An exceptionally high quantity and percentage of rapid eye movement (REM) sleep is present. REM sleep accounted for 224 min, or 50.1%, of total sleep time. This is close to 100% more than expected for a 31-year-old man. In light of the sudden reduction in dexedrine on the day before testing, this almost certainly is a massive REM sleep rebound. REM sleep latency also was short, at 9.0 min. Under other circumstances, this might be considered clinically significant. However, in the presence of a REM sleep rebound of this proportion, the short REM latency is not likely to have clinical significance.

9. A sleep efficiency of 96.7% is unusually high for a patient spending the first night in the sleep laboratory. The high sleep efficiency could be a result of previous sleep deprivation—the patient reported 6 hr of total sleep on the preceding night—or could be a function of the REM sleep rebound.

10. The patient reported sleeping better than usual. This strongly suggests that the quantity and quality of sleep are not typical for this patient. This must be taken into consideration before making any summary statements.

11. Sleep-disordered breathing is well within normal limits. The normal REM sleep related RDI is of special significance in light of the very high REM sleep percentage. Sleep disordered breathing typically is more severe during REM sleep.

12. The absence of snoring provides further support for the conclusion that sleep-disordered breathing is unlikely to contribute to the patient's symptoms.

13. The absence of significant numbers of arousing periodic leg movements in sleep (PLMS) also lends support to the theory that the patient's complaint is not secondary to a sleep-fragmenting disorder. However, it must also be taken into consideration that the massive REM sleep rebound might have interfered with the normal expression of PLMS. PLMS occurs almost exclusively during non-REM (NREM) sleep. Additionally, they most often appear during the first one third to one half of the sleep period, during a time when REM sleep predominated.

Sleep Histogram (Figure C3-3)

14. The histogram documents the massive REM sleep rebound that overwhelms normal sleep architecture.

Sample Interpretation

This recording is remarkable for the very high percentage of REM sleep and short REM sleep latency. A total of 224 min REM sleep were noted, for 50.1% of total sleep time. This extremely high percentage of REM sleep suggests the presence of rebound sleep. Rebound REM sleep can occur following a period of total sleep deprivation or partial cumulative sleep deprivation or withdrawal from alcohol and specific medications, such as tricyclic antidepressants, MAO inhibitors, and medication with anticholinergic properties. Additionally, a REM sleep rebound can result from a change in a sleep/wake rhythm or elimination of a sleep fragmenting process or sleep disorder. A review of the patient's questionnaires reveals that the patient had reduced his daily intake of dexedrine from 60 mg to 30 mg on the day of this sleep study. As dexedrine is a potent suppressor of REM sleep and sudden discontinuation of dexedrine is known to result in

Diagnostic Polysomnogram

Lights Out: 11:18 PM   **Lights On: 7:04 AM**

Sleep Parameters
General

	Minutes	% TRT	% TST	Latency	
Total Recording Time	463.0				
Total Sleep Time	447.5	96.7			
Total Wake Time	15.5	3.3			**7**
Stage 1 Sleep	25.0	5.4	5.6	7.0	
Stage 2 Sleep	160.0	34.6	35.8	0.0	
Stage 3 Sleep	21.0	4.5	4.7		
Stage 4 Sleep	17.5	3.8	3.9		
REM Sleep	224.0	48.4	50.1	9.0	**8**

Sleep Continuity Measures

Sleep Efficiency (%)	96.7	
Wake After Sleep Onset (Min)	15.5	**9**
# of Awakenings > 5 Minutes	0	
# of Awakenings > 1 Min & < 5 Min	18	
# of Arousals (all sources)	22.0	
Arousal Index (hr. of sleep)	2.9	

Patient Sleep Estimations

	Subjective	Objective
Total Sleep Time (hrs.)	7	7.5
Sleep Latency (mins.)	5	7.0
# of Awakenings	1	2

Patient Evaluation of Laboratory Sleep Compared to Usual Sleep

All in All:	Better than usual	**10**
AM Alertness:	Feel same as usual	

FIGURE C3-2
Polysomnogram (DPSG) report, page 1.

Sleep Disordered Breathing

	Obstructive Apneas		Hypopneas		Central Apneas				
	REM	NREM	REM	NREM	REM	NREM	REM	NREM	Total
#	0	0	6	5	1	1	7	6	13
Index	0.0	0.0	1.6	1.3	0.3	0.3	1.9	1.6	1.7
Average Duration	0	0	24	20	29	20			
Maximum Duration	0	0	34	27	29	20			
Average SaO2%	0	0	99	99	99	98			
Low SaO2%	0	0	98	98	99	98			

11

Body Position Effects

	Supine	Prone	Left	Right
Total Recording Time	229.0	0.0	0.0	190.5
Total Sleep Time	224.5	0.0	0.0	179.5
Sleep Efficiency	98.0	0.0	0.0	94.2
RDI	3.2	0.0	0.0	0.3
Low SaO2 %	98	0	0	99

Baseline Cardiorespiratory Parameters

	Wake		REM		NREM	
	High	Low	High	Low	High	Low
SaO2 (%)	100	99	100	99	100	99
Respiratory Rate	16	14	16	14	16	14
ECG	71	68	91	81	94	89

Other Cardiorespiratory Data

Snoring	None.
Cardiac Arrhythmia	None.
Undisturbed Sleep (hrs.)	1.0
Paradoxical Movements	None noted.

12

FIGURE C3-2
Polysomnogram (DPSG) report, page 2.

Movements in Sleep

Total Periodic Leg Movements in Sleep (PLMS)   43
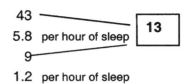
PLMS Index   5.8 per hour of sleep

Total Arousing PLMS   9

Arousing PLMS Index   1.2 per hour of sleep

Additional Findings

None.

Medication	Quantity	Time Taken
Ortho1	12 pm	
Dexedrine	5 mgs x 6	8 -12noon
Imitrex		

FIGURE C3-2
Polysomnogram (DPSG) report, page 3.

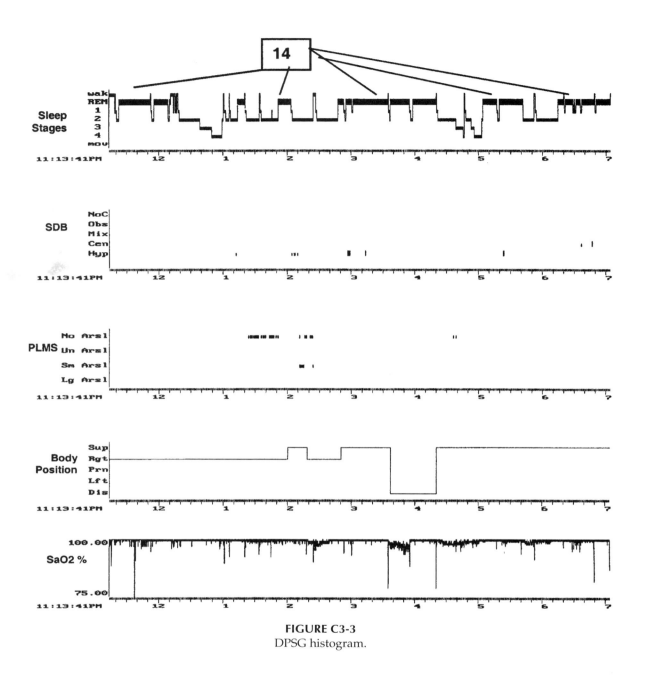

FIGURE C3-3
DPSG histogram.

REM sleep rebound, it is almost certain that the sudden reduction in dexedrine on the day of the study is the source of the high REM sleep percent. Latency to REM sleep generally is 90–120 minutes after sleep onset. The REM sleep latency of 9.0 min noted here was abnormally short. Under other circumstances, a REM sleep latency in this range could be suggestive of a diagnosis of narcolepsy or a major affective disorder or could be secondary to sleep deprivation or fragmentation or an irregular sleep/wake rhythm. However, in light of the massive sleep rebound noted, the short REM sleep latency is not suggestive of any specific sleep disorder.

Sleep apnea and other sleep-disordered breathing were not present during this recording. A small number of periodic leg movements in sleep were present in this recording but resulted in little sleep disruption. However, as PLMS generally are not present during REM sleep and REM sleep occupied an abnormally high percentage of total sleep time, PLMS may be more severe on nights with normal quantities of REM and NREM sleep.

Morning Questionnaire (Figure C3-4)

15. The patient reported sleeping better than usual. He also told the sleep technologist that the sleep laboratory was quieter than his bedroom at home. This suggests the possibility of an environmental sleep disorder. Better noise control, ear plugs, white noise machine, or the like might result in improvement in the subjective quality of sleep at home.

Multiple Sleep Latency Test (Figure C3-5)

The patient reported to technical staff that he had not taken any dexedrine on the day of the MSLT. Therefore, within two days he had discontinued 60 mg dexedrine.

16. The mean sleep latency of 0.8 min is within the range of severe daytime sleepiness. However, as withdrawal from amphetamines can be associated with daytime fatigue, these results cannot be considered valid.

17. The presence of three sleep-onset REM periods (SOREMPs) under other circumstances would be consistent with a diagnosis of narcolepsy. However, as sudden withdrawal from dexedrine clearly was associated with a massive REM sleep rebound during the prior night's sleep study and REM sleep rebound may continue for several days following withdrawal, these results cannot be considered valid support for the diagnosis of narcolepsy.

18. Conduct of a repeat MSLT should await complete withdrawal from medication for at least a week.

Sample Multiple Sleep Latency Test Interpretation

A mean sleep latency of 0.8 min (to stage 1 sleep) is consistent with the finding of severe daytime sleepiness. Under usual circumstances the presence of three sleep-onset REM periods would be consistent with a diagnosis of narcolepsy.

However, in light of the sudden discontinuation of dexedrine and the resulting massive rebound of REM sleep during the prior night (224 min, 50.1% of total sleep time) none of these results can be considered valid. The three SOREMPs can be the result of rebound REM sleep and therefore are not diagnostic of narcolepsy. The short mean sleep latency also cannot clearly be attributed to a sleep disorder in light of the well-known effects of amphetamine withdrawal. A repeat study with the patient off all analeptic medication for at least 10 days is indicated to properly rule out narcolepsy.

MORNING QUESTIONNAIRE

All things considered, your sleep last night was

(circle one answer)

1. Much better than usual
2. Better than usual
3. Same as usual
4. Worse than usual
5. Much worse than usual

Compared to the way you usually feel after awakening do you

1. Feel much more alert and awake than usual
2. Feel more alert and awake than usual
3. Feel same as usual
4. Feel less alert and awake than usual
5. Feel much less alert and wake than usual

How long did it take you to fall asleep last night? __5__ mins.

Compared to the usual time it takes you to fall asleep, this was
1. Much shorter
2. Shorter
3. Same
4. Longer
5. Much longer

How many hours/minutes did you sleep last night? ___7___ hrs./mins.

Compared to the usual time you sleep at home, this was
1. Much longer
2. Longer
3. Same
4. Shorter
5. Much shorter

How many times did you awaken last night? ___1___ times

Compared to the usual number of times your waken, this was
1. Many fewer than usual
2. Fewer than usual
3. Same
4. More than usual
5. Many more than usual

Please comment specifically on how your night in the sleep laboratory was different from sleep at home. _____

FIGURE C3-4
Morning questionnaire, page 1.

		Circle one	Describe
15	Room Temperature	Better ~~Same~~ Worse	_____
	~~Mattress~~	Better (Same) Worse	_____
	Pillow	Better (Same) Worse	_____
	Noise	(Better) Same Worse	_____
	Light	Better (Same Worse)	_____
	Sleeping Position	Better (Same Worse)	_____
	Blankets	Better (Same Worse)	_____
	Sense of Security	Better (Same) Worse	_____
	Snacks	Better (Same) Worse	_____
	TV	Better (Same) Worse	_____
	_____	Better Same Worse	_____
	_____	Better Same Worse	_____

In what way was your sleep or the sleeping environment better here than your bedroom at home? _____less noise_____

In what way was your sleep or the sleeping environment worse here than your bedroom at home? _____n/a_____

Did anything happen in the sleep laboratory (other than electrodes etc.) that does not usually happen at home?_____nothing_____

Does anything usually happen at home during sleep that did not happen here?
_____

How was the sleep test different from what you expected? _not different was ok_____

Any comments or suggestions? _____

FIGURE C3-4
Morning questionnaire, page 2.

MULTIPLE SLEEP LATENCY TEST (MSLT) REPORT

DESCRIPTION OF PROCEDURES: The MSLT consists of 4 twenty minute nap opportunities given at 2 hour intervals throughout the course of one day. Patients are instructed to fall asleep as quickly as possible. If sleep occurs the nap is terminated 15 minutes after sleep onset. Patients are not permitted to sleep between scheduled naps. All data are visually scored and analyzed according to standard criteria.

TEST RESULTS

16

LATENCIES (mins)					
	10:00 AM	12:00 PM	2:00 PM	4:00 PM	Mean
Latency to Stage 1	0.5	0.5	1.5	0.5	0.8
Latency to Stage 2	1.0	1.5	2.5	1.0	2.0
Latency to REM	2.0	2.5	12.0	-	-

17

MEDICATIONS: The patient reported decreasing her dosage of Dexedrine from 60 mg to 30 mg on the day before this study and completely discontinued all Dexedrine on the day of the study.

ADDITIONAL DATA: The patient reported that she was as alert as usual during the day. Technical staff reported that the patient had difficulty maintaining alertness in between naps.

18

FIGURE C3-5
MSLT report.

FINAL SYNTHESIS

The case points out the importance of knowing about and managing medication in patients scheduled for sleep studies.

FINAL NOTES

On receiving the DPSG and MSLT reports and cover letter, the referring physician forwarded a copy of his instructions to the patient. After completing his office consultation, the referring physician was very impressed with the severity of the patient's daytime sleepiness and the potential risk it represented. He immediately referred the patient for the diagnostic sleep studies, but due to high volume of referrals at the sleep laboratory, these could not be scheduled for 30 days. For this reason he prescribed 15 mg dexedrine spansules b.i.d. Additionally, he provided the patient an additional prescription for 5 mg dexedrine with instructions to take up to six per day, if necessary. He further instructed the patient to discontinue all dexedrine three to five days before testing. However, the patient was not provided a schedule for discontinuing medication and no one checked with the patient to assure compliance with the physician's orders.

Case 4

PRESENTING COMPLAINT

"I can't stay awake."

PATIENT DEMOGRAPHICS

The patient is a 35-year-old, married, white female biologist.

PATIENT SLEEP HISTORY

The patient reports a 10-year history of increasing daytime sleepiness. She is prone to doze off whenever physically inactive. She often feels sleepy while driving and has dozed off once. Two or three times weekly, she will pull off the road to take a short nap. She reports that these naps are refreshing but does not recall dreaming. She finds her sleepiness most severe after eating and especially after lunch in the 2–3 PM range.

The patient has no history suggestive of cataplexy, sleep paralysis, or hypnogogic hallucinations. She does not snore and has never awakened gasping for breathing or choking. However, she experiences nasal congestion related to seasonal allergies, and during those times, she will awaken with a dry mouth. The patient's husband reports hearing the sound of teeth grinding several times weekly.

She reports that her mother took occasional planned naps, but there is no family history suggestive of narcolepsy or sleep apnea.

The patient reports vivid dreams and nightmares two or three times per week.

SLEEP/WAKE SCHEDULE

The patient typically sleeps 4–5 hr on weeknights and 7–9 hr on weekends. She often awakens on weekdays feeling unrefreshed, while on weekends she often awakens feeling rested. She reports that, due to stress at work, she has awakened at 2 AM the last three Sunday nights, after only 2–3 hr of sleep. The awakenings occur during a vivid anxiety dream (nightmare), and she is unable to return to sleep thereafter. She takes no planned naps on days off but may doze off for 20–60 min while reading or watching TV. The patient typically awakens from sleep once nightly one or two times during the workweek and at least twice per night on the weekend.

MEDICAL HISTORY AND EXAM

On examination the patient is 5'3" and 112 lbs. Her blood pressure was 115/75 and pulse 56 and regular. Her ENT and neurological examinations were normal and her chest clear. Her only medication was birth control pills. She had taken no other prescription medications other than antibiotics for at least five years. The patient reports symptoms of temporal mandibular joint (TMJ) pain.

On interview she had no symptoms of depression although she was experiencing stress and anxiety related to her performance on a new job. She was especially concerned that her sleepiness would interfere with her ability to perform at a high level.

PRELIMINARY DIAGNOSES

1. Narcolepsy:
   Pro—Onset of sleepiness in early 20s, refreshing naps.
   Con—No cataplexy or other auxiliary symptoms.
2. Insufficient sleep:
   Pro—Weekday total sleep time of 4–5 hr and awakens unrefreshed, weekend total sleep time 7–9 hr and awakens refreshed.
3. Irregular Sleep/Wake schedule?
4. Transient insomnia:
   Pro—Experiences anticipatory anxiety Sunday nights.
5. Obstructive sleep apnea:
   Pro—Dry mouth in AM.
   Con—Thin, premenopausal woman who does not snore.
6. Bruxism.
7. Nightmares.

PLAN

1. Diagnostic polysomnogram (DPSG).
2. Multiple Sleep Latency Test (MSLT).

COMMENTARY ON CLINICAL MATERIALS

All boxed numbers in the figures refer to the following comments.

Sleep Log (Figure C4-1)

1. Patient dozes off several times weekly while watching TV. As these naps occur in the late evening, they appear to delay both lights out time and sleep onset.
2. Once asleep, the patient notes no long awakenings. Short awakenings, lasting seconds or even minutes, may be present but not perceived or remembered by the patient.
3. Total sleep time is extended to 9 hr or more on weekends compared to 5.5–6 hr on weekdays. However, the patient may take naps even after these relatively long sleep periods. This could sug-

gest that the patient's daytime sleepiness is not linked to the prior quantity of sleep. This would support a diagnosis of a sleep disorder not dependent on total sleep time such as narcolepsy. On the other hand, the weekend naps suggest that the 9–9.5 hr of sleep is insufficient to settle the sleep debt accumulated during weeknights.

4. The patient's overall fatigue ratings suggest high fatigue following shorter weeknight sleep periods and lower fatigue ratings following longer weekend sleep periods. This would support the theory that the patient's daytime sleepiness is secondary to cumulative partial sleep deprivation during the workweek that is only partially relieved by longer weekend sleep periods.

Bedtime Questionnaire (Figure C4-2)

5. This questionnaire documents a fairly typical weekday pattern of sleep on the night prior to the sleep study with sleep onset after midnight and 5–6 hr of total sleep time.

Diagnostic Polysomnogram (Figure C4-3)

6. The patient requested lights out at 10:23 PM, far earlier than any sleep time noted on the sleep log. The patient told the sleep technologist that the process of attaching electrodes and filling out the questionnaire prevented her from dozing off while watching TV. Latency to stage 1 sleep was only 4 min, suggesting the patient was quite sleepy.
7. The patient slept for 7.5 hr, slightly more than noted on the sleep log for a workday, but less than a weekend sleep period.
8. Sleep efficiency was very high, consistent with rebound sleep after sleep deprivation.
9. Stage 1 was slightly lower than expected, also consistent with rebound sleep as well as the absence of sleep fragmenting disorders such as sleep apnea or periodic leg movements in sleep.
10. Rapid eye movement (REM) sleep quantity and percentage were higher than expected, suggesting a REM sleep rebound. This may be consistent with the pattern of partial sleep deprivation noted on the sleep log but also could result from recent discontinuation of REM-suppressing medications or alcohol. It further is possible that the patient was self-medicating to compensate for her sleepiness. The sleep specialist should consider inquiring about this during the follow-up office visit.

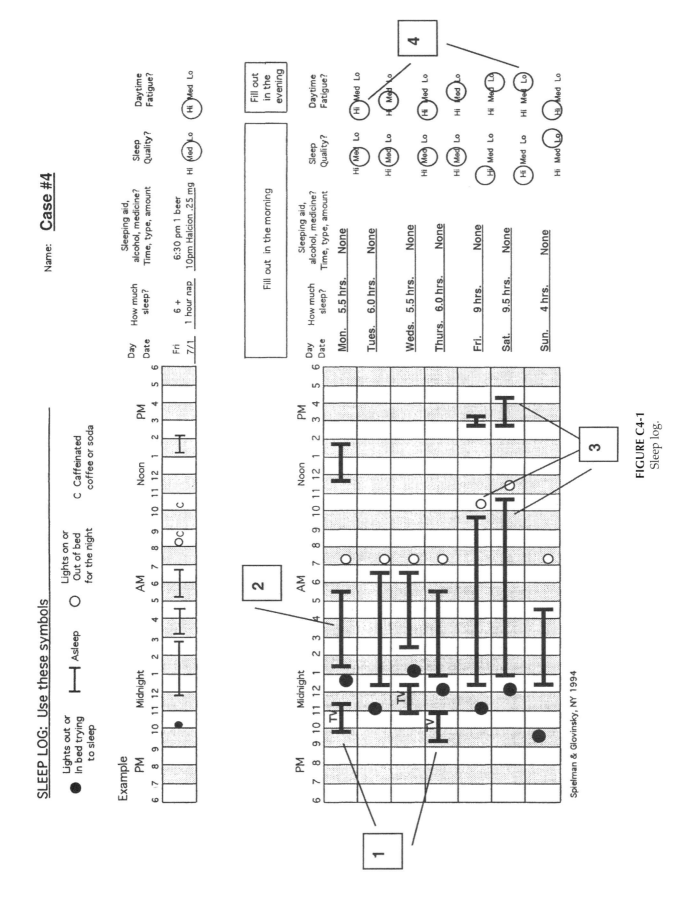

FIGURE C4-1
Sleep log.

Spielman & Glovinsky, NY 1994

127

BEDTIME QUESTIONNAIRE

How sleepy do you feel right now? Place mark along line.

Very sleepy_____✕_____ Very Alert

Please describe how you feel now. Circle one of the numbers on the Stanford Sleepiness Scale below:

1. Alert. Wide Awake. Energetic.
2. Functioning at a high level, but not at peak. Able to concentrate.
3. Awake, but not fully alert.
4. A little foggy, let down.
5. Foggy. Beginning to lose interest in remaining awake. Slowed down.
6. Cannot stay awake. Sleep onset soon.

Please describe your sleep last night:

What time did you turn out the lights?	About midnight , fell alseep with tv on
How long did it take to fall asleep?	_?___
How many hours/minutes did you sleep last night?	_5-6 hrs._
What time did you awaken this morning?	_6 AM
How many times did you awaken last night?	__0__

5

Did you nap or fall asleep today?   Yes   (No)
If YES, please indicate at what times and for how long
_____

Was today a typical day?   (Yes)   No
If NO, please explain
_____

How well do you expect to sleep tonight?
Very well _____

Do you feel ready to go to sleep right now?   (Yes)   No
If NO, please explain
_____

Did you drink any alcohol today?   (Yes)   No

If YES, please list what kind, how much and when taken
1 glass wine at 6 PM
_____

Did you drink any caffeinated beverages (coffee, tea, colas, etc.) today? YES (NO)

FIGURE C4-2
Bedtime questionnaire, page 1.

If YES, please what kind, when taken and how much?

_____

Did you smoke any cigarettes, cigars, pipe, etc. today?   (YES) NO

If YES, please what kind, when taken and how much?

_____

Please list all medications you took today. Be sure to include prescriptions medications as well as those you take without a prescription

Name	How Much	Reason	When Taken
None			

Please list any other medication you will be taking before going to sleep

Name	How Much	Reason	When Taken
None			

Please list any other medication you have stopped taking in the last 30 days.

Name	How Much	Reason	When Taken
Birth control			
Advil		Sinus Headache	

Please describe anything else that occurred last night or today that might affect your sleep tonight. _____

_____

FIGURE C4-2
Bedtime questionnaire, page 2.

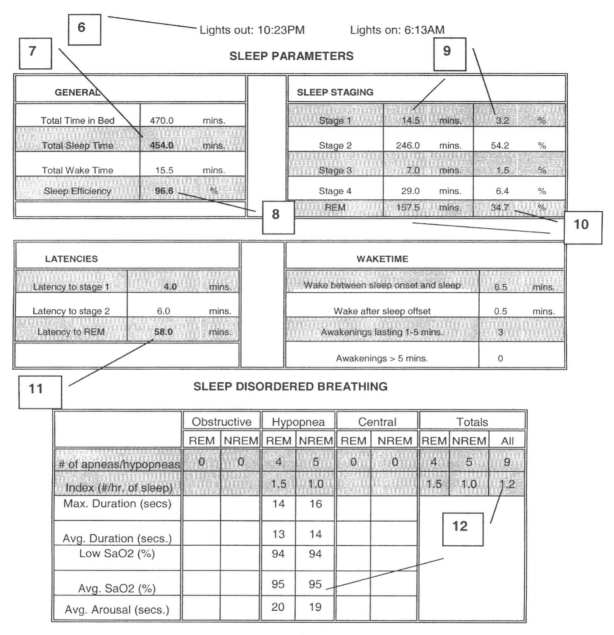

Lights out: 10:23PM   Lights on: 6:13AM

SLEEP PARAMETERS

GENERAL		
Total Time in Bed	470.0	mins.
Total Sleep Time	454.0	mins.
Total Wake Time	15.5	mins.
Sleep Efficiency	96.6	%

SLEEP STAGING			
Stage 1	14.5	mins.	3.2 %
Stage 2	246.0	mins.	54.2 %
Stage 3	7.0	mins.	1.5 %
Stage 4	29.0	mins.	6.4 %
REM	157.5	mins.	34.7 %

LATENCIES		
Latency to stage 1	4.0	mins.
Latency to stage 2	6.0	mins.
Latency to REM	58.0	mins.

WAKETIME		
Wake between sleep onset and sleep	6.5	mins.
Wake after sleep offset	0.5	mins.
Awakenings lasting 1-5 mins.	3	
Awakenings > 5 mins.	0	

SLEEP DISORDERED BREATHING

	Obstructive		Hypopnea		Central		Totals		
	REM	NREM	REM	NREM	REM	NREM	REM	NREM	All
# of apneas/hypopneas	0	0	4	5	0	0	4	5	9
Index (#/hr. of sleep)			1.5	1.0			1.5	1.0	1.2
Max. Duration (secs)			14	16					
Avg. Duration (secs.)			13	14					
Low SaO2 (%)			94	94					
Avg. SaO2 (%)			95	95					
Avg. Arousal (secs.)			20	19					

BASELINE CARDIORESPIRATORY DATA

	Wake	REM	NREM
ECG	73-99	56-73	50-67
Respiratory Rate	18-22	16-21	15-17
SaO2*	98-100 %	97-98 %	97-99 %

*SaO2 measured by pulse oximeter.

FIGURE C4-3
Polysomnogram (DPSG) report, page 1.

OTHER CARDIORESPIRATORY DATA

Body Position: The patient slept in the supine, prone and right lateral decubitus positions.

Undisturbed sleep: Approximately 4.5 hours.

Snoring: Rare snoring noted.

Arrhythmias: No cardiac arrhythmias noted.

MOVEMENT PARAMETERS

	#	Index
Total periodic leg movements in sleep (PLMS)	0	0 per hour of sleep
PLMS resulting in arousal		per hour of sleep
Duration of arousals		seconds
Total nonperiodic leg movements in sleep (NPLMS)	0	0 per hour of sleep
NPLMS resulting in arousal		per hour of sleep
Duration of arousals		seconds

ADDITIONAL FINDINGS

Paradoxical out-of-phase movements of the chest and abdomen were intermittently present when the patient slept in the supine position and while in REM sleep.

MEDICATIONS

Type	Amount	When taken

None noted by patient.

FIGURE C4-3
Polysomnogram (DPSG) report, page 2.

11. A REM sleep of 58 min is shorter than expected. It could occur simply as a function of the REM sleep rebound. However, REM sleep latencies in this range have been reported in depression. As the patient has reported significant job related stress, this explanation should be considered.

12. The diagnosis of sleep apnea can be ruled out, although rare snoring was confirmed.

Morning Questionnaire (Figure C4-4)

13. Despite the objective sleep data noted previously, the patient, for the most part, describes this night as typical.

14. Patient comments suggest poor sleep hygiene contributing to the pattern of falling asleep in late evening while reading or watching TV and then having to "wake up in order to go to sleep."

Sleep Histogram (Figure C4-5)

15. Sleep architecture is generally within normal limits except for the longer REM sleep duration and early REM sleep latency.

Sample Interpretation

This recording is remarkable for the absence of significant sleep-disordered breathing and changes in REM sleep quantity and timing. A total of nine hypopneas, partial obstructions of the upper airway, were noted for an overall respiratory disturbance index (RDI) of 1.2/hr of sleep. This is not considered abnormal. Hypopneas generally were short in duration, with the longest persisting for 16 sec. No significant snoring was noted throughout the recording. However, paradoxical movements of the chest and abdomen were noted occasionally, indicative of a partial obstruction of the upper airway during that time. Additionally, there were occasional arousals from sleep associated with K complexes that appeared consistent with a respiratory etiology, although none was evident. ECG was unremarkable.

The overall quality and quantity of sleep was generally good. Light stage 1 sleep was only slightly elevated and good quantities of deep sleep and REM sleep were noted. However, REM sleep was of sufficient quantity to be atypical or abnormal in two ways. REM sleep typically occurs 90–120 min after sleep onset. A REM sleep latency of 58 min, noted in this recording, is shorter than

expected. REM sleep latencies in this range have been reported to be associated with major affective disorders, circadian rhythm disorders, recent discontinuation of REM-sleep-suppressing medication, recent elimination of REM-sleep-fragmenting processes, or relief of recent acute or cumulative partial sleep deprivation. Additionally, the quantity and percentage of REM sleep in this recording is higher than expected for a patient of this age and most consistent with a REM sleep rebound. A REM sleep rebound could occur following discontinuation of a REM-sleep-suppressing medication (tricyclic antidepressants, MAO inhibitors, alcohol, etc.), following elimination of REM-sleep-fragmenting events (apneas, hypopneas, etc.), recent acute or chronic partial sleep deprivation, or a change in the usual sleep/wake schedule. A REM sleep rebound also could be the source of a short REM sleep latency as noted. The patient reported, on the AM questionnaire, sleeping the same as usual and awakening from sleep feeling as alert as usual.

In summary, these findings are not consistent with obstructive sleep apnea and changes in REM sleep are of uncertain significance.

Multiple Sleep Latency Test (Figure C4-6)

16. The patient failed to fall asleep on two occasions and had a very long sleep latency on a third nap. The failure to fall asleep on the final nap could be considered secondary to "cabin fever" and excluded from the mean sleep latency. However, the failure to sleep at the noon nap suggests that the patient may have normal alertness at certain times of the day. These results certainly are not consistent with significant daytime sleepiness of the type seen in narcolepsy or significant sleep apnea.

17. The mean sleep latency of 13.4 min is consistent with normal daytime alertness.

18. REM sleep was not present during any of the three naps during which sleep was recorded. The absence of REM sleep is inconsistent with diagnosis of narcolepsy but does not rule it out.

19. The technical staff followed standard MSLT protocols and had the patient stop all activity within 15 min of testing. However, the technologist noted that the patient was quite restless before both naps in which no sleep was recorded. As has been noted previously, physical activity prior to start of nap testing can significantly delay sleep onset. Care should be taken in interpretation when the patient is physically active prior to testing.

MORNING QUESTIONNAIRE

All things considered, your sleep last night was

(circle one answer)

1. Much better than usual
2. Better than usual
3. Same as usual
4. Worse than usual
5. Much worse than usual

Compared to the way you usually feel after awakening do you

1. Feel much more alert and awake than usual
2. Feel more alert and awake than usual
3. Feel same as usual
4. Feel less alert and awake than usual
5. Feel much less alert and wake than usual

How long did it take you to fall asleep last night? __20__ mins.

Compared to the usual time it takes you to fall asleep, this was
1. Much shorter
2. Shorter
3. Same
4. Longer
5. Much longer

How many hours/minutes did you sleep last night? __7.5__ hrs./mins.

Compared to the usual time you sleep at home, this was
1. Much longer
2. Longer
3. Same
4. Shorter
5. Much shorter

How many times did you awaken last night? __2-3__ times

Compared to the usual number of times your waken, this was
1. Many fewer than usual
2. Fewer than usual
3. Same
4. More than usual
5. Many more than usual

$\boxed{13}$

FIGURE C4-4
Morning questionnaire, page 1.

Please comment specifically on how your night in the sleep laboratory was different from sleep at home

	Circle one	Describe
Room Temperature	Better (Same) Worse	_____
Mattress	Better Same Worse	_____
Pillow	Better (Same) Worse	_____
Noise	~~Better~~ Same (Worse)	could hear talking
Light	(Better) Same Worse	_____
Sleeping Position	Better Same (Worse)	Electrodes, etc
Blankets	Better (Same) Worse	_____
Sense of Security	Better (Same) Worse	_____
Snacks	Better (Same) Worse	_____
TV	Better (Same) Worse	_____
_____	Better Same Worse	_____
_____	Better Same Worse	_____

In what way was your sleep or the sleeping environment better here than your bedroom at home? _Got into bed on purpose instead of dozing off in from of TV or while reading and getting into be later_

14

In what way was your sleep or the sleeping environment worse here than your bedroom at home? _Not bad at all, just restricted initially by electrodes_

Did anything happen in the sleep laboratory (other than electrodes etc.) that does not usually happen at home?_ Nothing._

Does anything usually happen at home during sleep that did not happen here? Usually dream more and may awaken from dreams, also I am told I grind my teeth.

How was the sleep test different from what you expected? _More electrodes than I expected, but other wise no problem_

Any comments or suggestions? _____

FIGURE C4-4
Morning questionnaire, page 2.

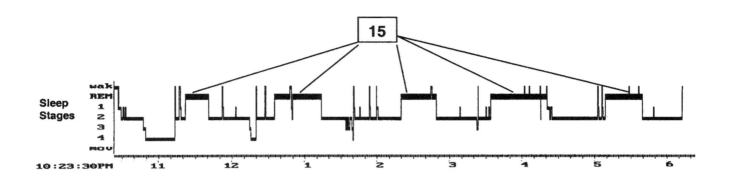

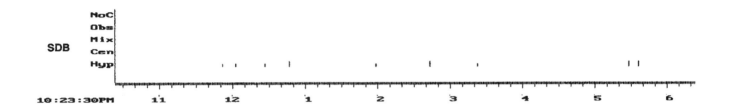

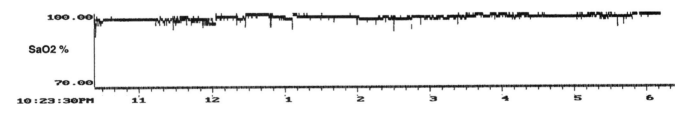

FIGURE C4-5
Polysomnogram (DPSG) histogram.

MULTIPLE SLEEP LATENCY TEST (MSLT) REPORT

DESCRIPTION OF PROCEDURES: The MSLT consists of 5 twenty minute nap opportunities given at 2 hour intervals throughout the course of one day. Patients are instructed to fall asleep as quickly as possible. If sleep occurs the nap is terminated 15 minutes after sleep onset. Patients are not permitted to sleep between scheduled naps. All data are visually scored and analyzed according to standard criteria.

TEST RESULTS

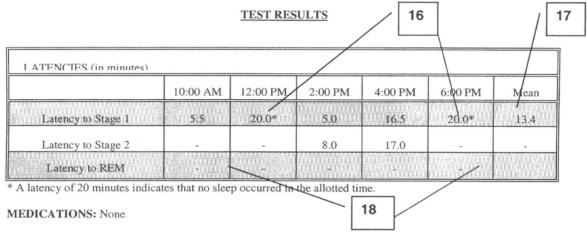

LATENCIES (in minutes)						
	10:00 AM	12:00 PM	2:00 PM	4:00 PM	6:00 PM	Mean
Latency to Stage 1	5.5	20.0*	5.0	16.5	20.0*	13.4
Latency to Stage 2	-	-	8.0	17.0	-	-
Latency to REM	-	-	-	-	-	-

* A latency of 20 minutes indicates that no sleep occurred in the allotted time.

MEDICATIONS: None

ADDITIONAL DATA: The patient reported that she was as alert as usual during the day. Patient was restless prior to naps at noon, 2 PM and 6 PM. Prior to those naps she paced the hallway outside of her sleep room.

FIGURE C4-6
MSLT report.

Sample Interpretation

A mean sleep latency of 13.4 min (to stage 1 sleep) is consistent with the finding of normal daytime alertness. However, there was considerable variation across the day, with the latencies at 10 AM and 2 PM reflecting significant and possibly abnormal sleepiness, while no sleep was noted at noon and 6 PM. The absence of sleep at 6 PM often is thought to reflect anxiety to finish the 20 hr period of testing and not the patient's actual level of alertness. The absence of REM sleep in this study is not supportive of a diagnosis of narcolepsy.

In summary, these findings are consistent with normal daytime alertness.

FINAL SYNTHESIS

The diagnostic polysomnogram and MLST were successful in ruling out narcolepsy and sleep apnea, thus narrowing the field of potential diagnoses. The sleep log, diagnostic polysomnogram, and MSLT lend significant support to the diagnosis of insufficient sleep as the source of the patient's daytime complaints. The insufficient sleep, in turn, would be secondary to cumulative partial sleep deprivation due to poor sleep hygiene, sleep/wake schedule problems, and transient anxiety-related insomnia. The patient's history further suggests the dream anxiety attacks (nightmares) and bruxism might contribute to sleep maintenance problems.

Case 5

PATIENT DEMOGRAPHICS

The patient is a 40-year-old, single mother of two girls. Trained as an accountant, she currently is at home with her children.

PATIENT SLEEP HISTORY

The patient has been snoring since age 16 years. Currently she awakens three or four times a night from a snore or to find herself gasping for breath. She also notes that, on awakening, she experiences palpitations, dry mouth, and often a headache. Additionally, she describes vivid dreams. She sleeps with one of her daughters, who is instructed to awaken her if she stops breathing. This occurs, on average, three or four times nightly. The patient reports getting into bed between 10:30 and 11 PM and attempts to awaken at 6:30 AM to get her children ready for school. She describes extreme difficulty awakening fully, with her children making repeated attempts to get her out of bed.

The patient describes herself as extremely sleepy for over 20 years. She has fallen asleep while driving, eating, talking, and at work. She cites her severe daytime sleepiness as the main reason for her very poor work record. The patient denies any symptoms consistent with cataplexy, sleep paralysis, or hypnogogic halluci-

nations. Family history is negative for any complaints of daytime sleepiness or other symptoms of narcolepsy.

The patient reports napping twice weekly, each time for 2 hr, with naps beginning shortly after lunchtime.

MEDICAL HISTORY AND EXAM

The patient is 5'6" and weighs 225 lbs. The patient has gained 60 lbs over the last 10 years and 30 lbs in the last six months. Her medical history is remarkable for lifelong menstrual difficulties. She reports only two to four menstrual periods yearly. A consultation with an endocrinologist at age 18 resulted in a diagnosis of "severe hormonal problems." However, she has not received treatment for these problems. Her medical history and physical examination otherwise were unremarkable.

PRELIMINARY DIAGNOSES

1. Obstructive sleep apnea:
   Pro—
   • Long history of snoring.
   • Nightly snore-related arousals.
   • Nightly arousals with gasping.
   • Nightly witnessed apneas.
   • AM dry mouth.
   • AM headache.
   • Unrefreshing sleep.
   • AM grogginess.
   • Severe daytime sleepiness.
   • Recent significant weight gain.

Con—
- Onset of sleepiness in early 20s.
- Premenopausal? Patient's history of menstrual and hormonal difficulties may permit onset of symptoms typical for postmenopausal women.
2. Narcolepsy
  Pro—Early onset of sleepiness, vivid dreams.
  Con—See preceding.

PLAN

1. Diagnostic polysomnogram (DPSG).
2. Multiple Sleep Latency Test (MSLT).

COMMENTARY ON CLINICAL MATERIALS

All boxed numbers on the figures refer to the comments that follow.

Sleep Log

The patient did not provide a sleep log, as requested. In this case, it would have been useful in scheduling the DPSG and MSLT at times appropriate for the patient.

Bedtime Questionnaire (Figure C5-1)

1. The patient reported taking 90 min to fall asleep on the previous night. This is at odds with the history she provided.
2. The patient previously stated that she took naps twice weekly. Nevertheless, she described the day before testing as atypical because she did not take a nap.

Diagnostic Polysomnogram (Figure C5-2)

3. The quantity and quality of sleep recorded is better than her history suggests.
4. The quantity and percentage of REM sleep is much higher than expected in a patient of this age, especially in light of expected sleep fragmentation secondary to sleep apnea. It is suggestive of REM sleep rebound from an unknown source.
5. Sleep-disordered breathing is within normal limits in all respects except for loud snoring. Based on the extensive list of symptoms suggestive of sleep apnea, these findings are unexpected.

6. Loud snoring was present in all sleep positions.
7. The patient deviated from her usual sleeping habits by elevating her head and upper body with two large pillows. Even minor changes in bedtime routine can have unexpected and sometimes major effects on sleep parameters.

Sleep Histogram (Figure C5-3)

8. Sleep architecture is consistent with not only rebound REM sleep but also rebound deep sleep. No major periods of wakefulness are present.

Sample Interpretation

This recording is remarkable for the absence of significant sleep-disordered breathing and the unusual sleep patterns. A total of only 26 apneas and hypopneas were recorded during 7.1 hr of sleep, for an overall respiratory disturbance index (RDI) of 3.7/hr of sleep. Although this number is more than usually reported in premenopausal women, it is less than the RDI of five or more per hour required for the clinical diagnosis of sleep apnea. However, loud snoring was noted in all sleep positions.

The overall quantity and quality of sleep was better than expected. Rapid eye movement (REM) sleep accounted for 41% of total sleep time, significantly more than the 15–25% expected in a woman of this age. This high percentage of REM sleep is consistent with a REM sleep rebound. REM sleep rebound may occur when a sleep fragmenting process such as sleep apnea is reduced or eliminated. This recording provided no evidence of severe sleep apnea. However, the patient changed her usual bedtime routine by sleeping on two large pillows. Elevation of the head can result in a treatment effect and reduce the frequency of apneas and hypopneas. Therefore, it is possible that raising her head resulted in accidental treatment of the patient's sleep apnea. Alternately, REM sleep rebounds of this degree can occur following discontinuation of REM-sleep-suppressing medications. However, the patient denies use of medication that might have such an effect.

This recording provides no direct evidence of sleep apnea. However, the unusual sleep findings suggest that the study should be repeated with strict adherence to the patient's usual bedtime routine and habits.

BEDTIME QUESTIONNAIRE

How sleepy do you feel right now? Place mark along line.

Very sleepy_____ Very Alert

Please describe how you feel now. Circle one of the numbers on the Stanford Sleepiness Scale below:

1. Alert. Wide Awake. Energetic.
2. Functioning at a high level, but not at peak. Able to concentrate.
3. Awake, but not fully alert.
4. A little foggy, let down.
5. Foggy. Beginning to lose interest in remaining awake. Slowed down.
6. Cannot stay awake. Sleep onset soon.

Please describe your sleep last night:

What time did you turn out the lights?	11:30 PM	
How long did it take to fall asleep?	90 minutes	
How many hours/minutes did you sleep last night?	6 hours	1
What time did you awaken this morning?	6:30 AM	
How many times did you awaken last night?	2	

Did you nap or fall asleep today?   Yes   No
If YES, please indicate at what times and for how long

_____   2

Was today a typical day?   Yes   No
If NO, please explain
I didn't take a nap today.

How well do you expect to sleep tonight?

Very Well.

Do you feel ready to go to sleep right now?   Yes   No
If NO, please explain
I feel tired, but not ready to go to bed.

Did you drink any alcohol today?   Yes   No

If YES, please list what kind, how much and when taken

FIGURE C5-1
Bedtime questionnaire, page 1.

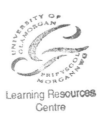

Did you drink any caffeinated beverages (coffee, tea, colas, etc.) today? YES **NO**

If YES, please what kind, when taken and how much?

_____

Did you smoke any cigarettes, cigars, pipe, etc. today?   YES **NO**

If YES, please what kind, when taken and how much?

_____

Please list all medications you took today. Be sure to include prescriptions medications as well as those you take without a prescription

Name	How Much	Reason	When Taken
None			

Please list any other medication you will be taking before going to sleep

Name	How Much	Reason	When Taken
None			

Please list any other medication you have stopped taking in the last 30 days.

Name	How Much	Reason	When Taken
None			

Please describe anything else that occurred last night or today that might affect your sleep tonight.

_____

FIGURE C5-1
Bedtime questionnaire, page 2.

SLEEP PARAMETERS

Lights off: 11:34 PM   Lights on: 7:02 AM

<u>General:</u>
Total Time in Bed: 446.5 mins.
Total Sleep Time: 426.5 mins. **3**
Total Waketime: 20.0 mins.
Sleep Efficiency: 95.5 %

<u>Latencies:</u>
Sleep latency (st.1):   15.0 mins.
Sleep latency (st.2):   17.5 mins.
REM latency: 64.5 mins.

<u>Sleep staging:</u>
stage 1: 11.0 mins. 2.6 %
stage 2: 172.5 mins. 40.4 %
stage 3: 37.0 mins. 8.7 %
stage 4: 27.5 mins. 6.4 %
REM: 178.5 mins. 41.9 %

4

<u>Waketime:</u>
Wake between sleep onset
 and sleep offset: 19.5 mins.
Wake after sleep offset: 0.5 mins.
Awakenings lasting 1-5 minutes: 1
Awakenings > 5 minutes: 0

RESPIRATORY PARAMETERS

	Obstructive		Hypopnea		Central		Totals		
	REM	NREM	REM	NREM	REM	NREM	REM	NREM	ALL
# of events:	0	5	8	7	6	0	14	11	26
Index (#/hr. of sleep):	0	0.7	1.1	1.0	0.8	0	4.7	2.6	3.7
Max. Duration (secs.):	–	25	18	18	18	–			
Avg. Duration (secs.):	–	19	14	14	14	–			
Low SaO2 (%):	–	92	93	93	93	–			
Avg. SaO2 (%):	–	94	98	97	98	–			
Avg. arousal (secs.)	–	14	6	4	3	–			

5

OTHER CARDIORESPIRATORY DATA

Baseline	Wake	REM	NREM
ECG	68-84	54-77	60-76
Respiratory rate:	16-20	16-22	14-18
SaO2*:	99-100%	99-100%	99-100%

<u>Body Position:</u> The patient slept supine, and left lateral decubitus.
<u>Post apnea/hypopnea arousals:</u> Usually ranged 3 - 25 seconds.
<u>Undisturbed sleep:</u> Approximately 7 hours were recorded while in both   **6**
positions during all stages of sleep.
<u>Snoring:</u> Was continuous, very loud and rhythmic while in the non-supine
position, and loud and intermittent while supine.
<u>Arrhythmias:</u> None.
<u>Misc.:</u> The patient slept on two thick pillows, instead of her usual 1 thin
        pillow.
7

*SaO2 measured by pulse oximetry.

FIGURE C5-2
Polysomnogram (DPSG) report.

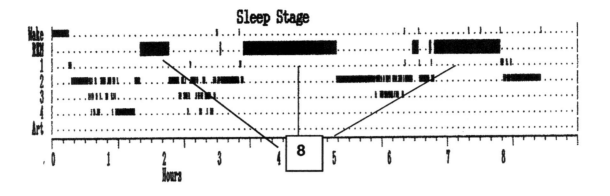

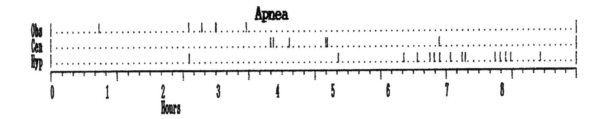

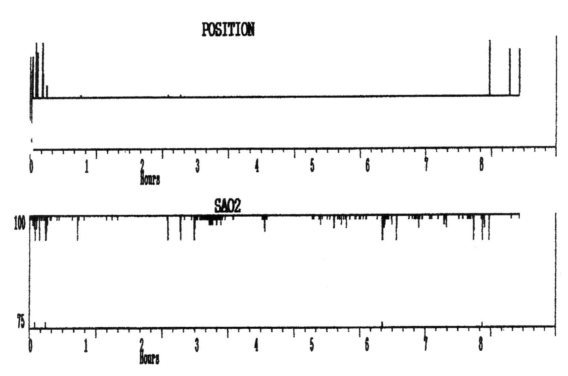

FIGURE C5-3
Polysomnogram (DPSG) histogram.

Morning Questionnaire (Figure C5-4)

9. Consistent with the results of the polysomnogram, the patient reports that she slept better than usual in the sleep laboratory.

10. She specifies that she fell asleep faster, slept longer, and did not awaken at all. These responses, along with the objective sleep parameters, confirm that this night of sleep was not typical of the patient's sleep at home in any respect.

Multiple Sleep Latency Test (Figure C5-5)

11. The patient failed to fall asleep on three occasions.

12. The mean sleep latency of 14.7 min is consistent with normal daytime alertness and inconsistent with the patient's description of disabling daily daytime sleepiness.

13. REM sleep is absence. The absence of sleep-onset REM periods (SOREMPs) is inconsistent with the diagnosis of narcolepsy but does not rule it out.

Note: In light of the high likelihood that the results of the diagnostic polysomnogram were not typical of the patient's sleep at home and instead represented an accidental treatment effect, another diagnostic polysomnogram was conducted.

Repeat Diagnostic Polysomnogram (Figure C5-6)

14. Total sleep time and sleep efficiency were reduced compared to the first sleep study. Generally, it is expected that sleep time and sleep quality will improve on the second night in the sleep laboratory compared with the first night.

15. Sleep fragmentation, as measured by stage 1 sleep, increased dramatically from 2.6% on the first sleep study to 29.3% on the second sleep study.

16. The number of awakenings increased significantly as well, with awakenings lasting more than 5 min—those most likely to be recalled by the patient—increasing from none to six.

17. Severe obstructive sleep apnea is now present, with an RDI of 42.8/hr of sleep and a low SaO_2 of 79%.

18. Great care was taken to make sure the patient slept in her usual body positions and with only one pillow. To be certain, she was asked to bring her own pillow from home.

19. Cardiac arrhythmias were present in this study that had not been noted in the first study. Eight episodes of second-degree AV blocks, with durations of 1–5 sec each, were noted to occur during REM-sleep-related obstructive apneas.

Repeat Diagnostic Polysomnogram Histogram (Figure C5-7)

20. Sleep was highly fragmented, with numerous short and long awakenings.

21. Significant hypoxia was noted, most severe during REM sleep.

Sample Interpretation

This recording is remarkable for the sleep-disordered breathing and cardiac arrhythmias. A total of 279 apneas and hypopneas were noted during 6.5 hr of sleep for an overall respiratory disturbance index of 42.8/hr of sleep. Apneas and hypopneas were associated with significant decreases in SaO_2 with 79% the lowest SaO_2 recorded. Apneas and hypopneas during REM sleep were associated with both first- and second-degree AV block, lasting 1–5 sec each. These arrhythmias most often occurred at the end of REM-sleep-related obstructive apneas with significant hypoxia. Loud snoring was heard throughout the recording in all sleep positions and all sleep stages.

The quantity and quality of sleep was poor. Light stage 1 sleep accounted for 24% of total sleep time, while deep sleep accounted for only 4.9% of total sleep time. In addition to the elevated percentage of light stage 1 sleep, all episodes of sleep-disordered breathing were associated brief arousals from sleep, lasting 5–10 sec, that may not be represented in the standard sleep parameters. The patient reported that her sleep was typical of her sleep at home.

In summary, this recording is consistent with a diagnosis of severe obstructive sleep apnea.

Note: With severe obstructive sleep apnea now confirmed polysomnograpically, the patient returned for a treatment trial of continuous positive airway pressure (CPAP).

MORNING QUESTIONNAIRE

All things considered, your sleep last night was

(circle one answer)

1. Much better than usual
2. Better than usual
3. Same as usual
4. Worse than usual
5. Much worse than usual

Compared to the way you usually feel after awakening do you

1. Feel much more alert and awake than usual
2. Feel more alert and awake than usual
3. Feel same as usual
4. Feel less alert and awake than usual
5. Feel much less alert and wake than usual

9

How long did it take you to fall asleep last night? 15 mins.

Compared to the usual time it takes you to fall asleep, this was
1. Much shorter
2. Shorter
3. Same
4. Longer
5. Much longer

How many hours/minutes did you sleep last night? _7 hrs./ 15 mins_

Compared to the usual time you sleep at home, this was
1. Much longer
2. Longer
3. Same
4. Shorter
5. Much shorter

How many times did you awaken last night? _0 times_

10

Compared to the usual number of times your waken, this was
1. Many fewer than usual
2. Fewer than usual
3. Same
4. More than usual
5. Many more than usual

FIGURE C5-4
Morning questionnaire.

DESCRIPTION OF PROCEDURES: The MSLT consists of 4-5 twenty minute nap opportunities given at 2 hour intervals throughout the course of one day. If sleep occurs the nap is terminated 15 minutes after sleep onset. Patients are not permitted to sleep between scheduled naps. All data are visually scored and analyzed according to standard criteria.

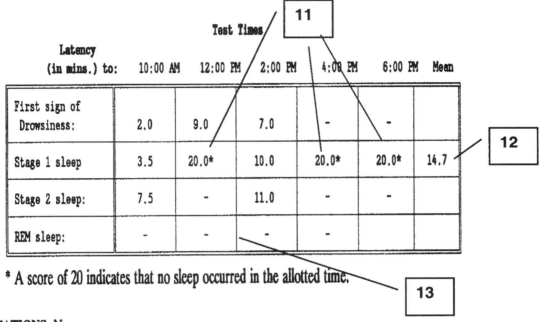

Test Times

Latency (in mins.) to:	10:00 AM	12:00 PM	2:00 PM	4:00 PM	6:00 PM	Mean
First sign of Drowsiness:	2.0	9.0	7.0	-	-	
Stage 1 sleep	3.5	20.0*	10.0	20.0*	20.0*	14.7
Stage 2 sleep:	7.5	-	11.0	-	-	
REM sleep:	-	-	-	-	-	

11

12

13

* A score of 20 indicates that no sleep occurred in the allotted time.

MEDICATIONS: None

FIGURE C5-5
MSLT report.

SLEEP PARAMETERS

Lights off: 10:02 PM Lights on: 5:55 AM

General:
  Total Time in Bed: 472.0 mins.
  Total Sleep Time: 391.0 mins.
  Total Waketime: 81.5 mins.
  Sleep Efficiency: 82.8 %

14

Latencies:
  Sleep latency (st.1):   1.0 mins.
  Sleep latency (st.2):   2.0 mins.
  REM latency: 102.0 mins.

Sleep staging:
  stage 1: 114.5 mins. 29.3 %
  stage 2: 225.5 mins. 57.7 %
  stage 3: 15.5 mins. 4.0 %
  stage 4:   7.5 mins. 1.9 %
  REM: 28.0 mins. 7.2 %

15

Waketime:
  Wake between sleep onset
   and sleep offset: 76.5 mins.
  Wake after sleep offset: 4.0 mins.
  Awakenings lasting 1-5 minutes: 13
  Awakenings > 5 minutes: 6

16

RESPIRATORY PARAMETERS

	Obstructive		Hypopnea		Central		Totals		
	REM	NREM	REM	NREM	REM	NREM	REM	NREM	ALL
# of events:	17	55	24	183	0	0	41	207	279
Index (#/hr. of sleep):	34	9	48	30	0	0	82	34	42.8
Max. Duration (secs.):	33	27	31	31	-	-			
Avg. Duration (secs.):	25	27	20	19	-	-			
Low SaO2 (%):	79	83	82	85	-	-			
Avg. SaO2 (%):	89	90	89	90	-	-			
Avg. arousal (secs.)	9	16	6	20	-	-			

17

OTHER CARDIORESPIRATORY DATA

Baseline	Wake	REM	NREM
ECG	84-98	56-91	52-91
Respiratory rate:	14-20	24-40	18-28
SaO2*:	97-100%	88-100% **	96-98 %

Body Position: The patient slept supine, and left and right lateral decubitus
        with and without 1 flat pillow.
Post apnea/hypopnea arousals: Ranged 3 seconds to 6.5 minutes.
Undisturbed sleep: Approximately 2.0 hours were recorded while in NREM sleep.
Snoring: Very loud, continuous and rhythmic, and occurred while in all
        positions and during all stage slept.
Arrhythmias: First degree and second degree AV block during REM sleep-related
        apneas.

18

19

*SaO2 measured by pulse oximetry.
**Represents resaturation values due to no respiratory event-free REM sleep.

FIGURE C5-6
Repeat polysomnogram (DPSG) report.

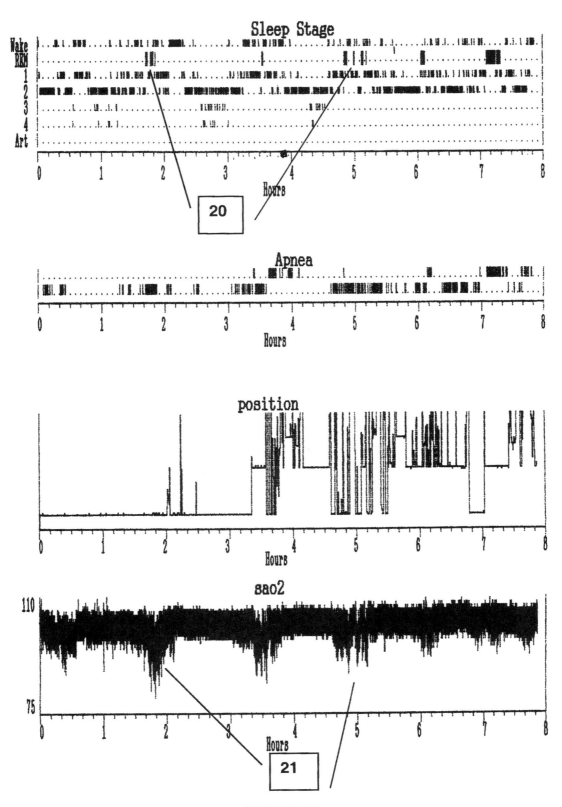

FIGURE C5-7
Repeat DPSG histogram.

Pre-Continuous Positive Airway Pressure Bedtime Questionnaire (Figure C5-8)

22. The patient reports a typical night of sleep, with 4.5 hr of total sleep time and three naps on the day prior to the CPAP recording.

Continuous Positive Airway Pressure Treatment Trial Results (Figures C5-9 and C5-10)

23. With administration of CPAP, stage 1 sleep was reduced to near normal limits.

24. REM sleep and deep sleep increased to the normal range but did not show the dramatic rebound noted on the first diagnostic sleep study. Is it possible that the sleep depth was higher prior to the first sleep study and therefore resulted in increased rebound compared to the second study? This is far from certain.

25. Although all pressures administered resulted in significant reduction or elimination of classically defined apneas and hypopneas, lower pressures did not result in elimination of snoring and paradoxical breathing. A pressure of 10 cm H_2O was determined to be optimal, in that it had the greatest effects at the lowest pressure.

26. The patient slept the entire recording in the supine position. This made it relatively easy to titrate pressure under the worst conditions: a supine position during REM sleep.

27. The goal of pressure titration is to reduce sleep-disordered breathing of all types.

28. A single episode of AV block persisted, even during CPAP.

29. The patient described her sleep as much better than usual and awoke feeling much more alert than usual. The subjective response of the patient may be as important or more important than objective measures that show improvement.

30. All subjective aspects of sleep were improved. Additionally, she told the sleep technologist that she could not remember being this alert "ever" and felt much better than after the first diagnostic sleep study.

Sample Interpretation

Administration of CPAP at a pressure of 10 cm H_2O resulted in a change from a respiratory disturbance index of 42.8/hr of sleep to an index of 1.1/hr of sleep. This is consistent with a change from severe obstructive sleep apnea to the normal respiration of sleep. The quality of sleep improved significantly, with light, stage 1 sleep reduced 29.3% to 9%. Additionally, deep sleep and REM sleep increased significantly. The patient reported that she slept much better than usual and awoke feeling more alert than usual. ECG was generally normal throughout the recording, except for one brief episode of REM-sleep-related AV block.

BEDTIME QUESTIONNAIRE

How sleepy do you feel right now? Place mark along line.

Very sleepy_____✕_____ Very Alert

Please describe how you feel now. Circle one of the numbers on the Stanford Sleepiness Scale below:

1. Alert. Wide Awake. Energetic.
2. Functioning at a high level, but not at peak. Able to concentrate.
3. Awake, but not fully alert.
4. A little foggy, let down.
5. Foggy. Beginning to lose interest in remaining awake. Slowed down.
6. Cannot stay awake. Sleep onset soon.

Please describe your sleep last night:

What time did you turn out the lights?	10:30 PM
How long did it take to fall asleep?	10 mins
How many hours/minutes did you sleep last night?	4.5 hours
What time did you awaken this morning?	7:15 AM
How many times did you awaken last night?	3

22

Did you nap or fall asleep today?   Yes   No
If YES, please indicate at what times and for how long
2 PM for 30 mins, 6 PM for 25 mins., 9:45 PM for 15 mins.

Was today a typical day?   Yes   No
If NO, please explain

_____

How well do you expect to sleep tonight?
Hopefully better
_____

Do you feel ready to go to sleep right now?   Yes   No
If NO, please explain
_____

Did you drink any alcohol today?   Yes   No

If YES, please list what kind, how much and when taken
_____

Did you drink any caffeinated beverages (coffee, tea, colas, etc.) today? YES NO

FIGURE C5-8
Pre-CPAP PM questionnaire, page 1.

If YES, please what kind, when taken and how much?

_____

Did you smoke any cigarettes, cigars, pipe, etc. today?   YES (NO)

If YES, please what kind, when taken and how much?

_____

Please list all medications you took today. Be sure to include prescriptions
medications as well as those you take without a prescription

Name	How Much	Reason	When Taken
None	_____	_____	_____
_____	_____	_____	_____
_____	_____	_____	_____
_____	_____	_____	_____
_____	_____	_____	_____
_____	_____	_____	_____
_____	_____	_____	_____

Please list any other medication you will be taking before going to sleep

Name	How Much	Reason	When Taken
None____	_____	_____	_____
_____	_____	_____	_____
_____	_____	_____	_____
_____	_____	_____	_____
_____	_____	_____	_____

Please list any other medication you have stopped taking in the last 30 days.

Name	How Much	Reason	When Taken
None____	_____	_____	_____
_____	_____	_____	_____
_____	_____	_____	_____

Please describe anything else that occurred last night or today that might affect
your sleep tonight.
_Nothing_____

FIGURE C5-8
Pre-CPAP PM questionnaire, page 2.

Lights out: 12:19 AM   Lights on: 7:40 AM

SLEEP PARAMETERS

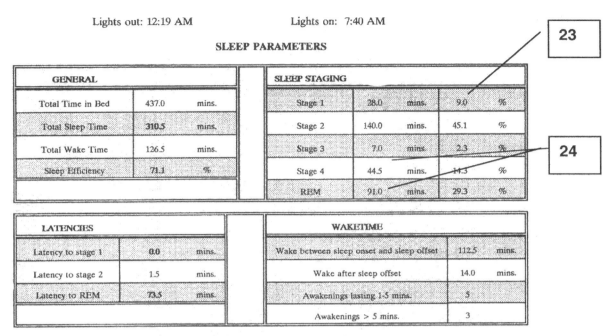

GENERAL		
Total Time in Bed	437.0	mins.
Total Sleep Time	310.5	mins.
Total Wake Time	126.5	mins.
Sleep Efficiency	71.1	%

SLEEP STAGING				
Stage 1	28.0	mins.	9.0	%
Stage 2	140.0	mins.	45.1	%
Stage 3	7.0	mins.	2.3	%
Stage 4	44.5	mins.	14.3	%
REM	91.0	mins.	29.3	%

23

24

LATENCIES		
Latency to stage 1	0.0	mins.
Latency to stage 2	1.5	mins.
Latency to REM	73.5	mins.

WAKETIME		
Wake between sleep onset and sleep offset	112.5	mins.
Wake after sleep offset	14.0	mins.
Awakenings lasting 1-5 mins.	5	
Awakenings > 5 mins.	3	

SLEEP DISORDERED BREATHING
(by CPAP pressure level)

Pressure Level in cm. H2O	Total Time Pressure Administered (mins.)	Index of Obstructive Apneas (per hour of sleep)	Index of Hypopneas (per hour of sleep)	Index of Central Apneas (per hour of sleep)	Total Apnea/Hypopnea Index (per hour of sleep)
No Pressure	0.0	0.0	0.0	0.0	0.0
5.0	21.5	0.0	2.5	0.0	2.5
7.5	12.5	0.0	0.0	0.0	0.0
10.0	276.5	0.0	0.7	0.4	1.1
12.5	0.0	0.0	0.0	0.0	0.0
15.0	0.0	0.0	0.0	0.0	0.0
17.5	0.0	0.0	0.0	0.0	0.0

25

ADDITIONAL NCPAP DATA

NCPAP was administered initially with a pressure of 5 cm H2O. This eliminated most respiratory events and reduced the volume of snoring. Administration of a pressure of 7.5 cm H2O further reduced the volume of snoring. Snoring was eliminated with a pressure of 10 cm H2O.

FIGURE C5-9
CPAP report, page 1.

BASELINE CARDIORESPIRATORY DATA

	Wake	REM	NREM
ECG	68-88	64-72	68-81
Respiratory Rate	12-15	16-18	16-19
SaO2*	99-100 %	99-100 %	98-100 %

*SaO2 measured by pulse oximeter.

OTHER CARDIORESPIRATORY DATA

Body Position: Sleep was recorded while in the supine position. ⟶ 26
Post Apnea/hypopnea arousals: Averaged 15 seconds.
Undisturbed sleep: Approximately 3.5 hours.
Snoring: Was eliminated with 10 cm H2O. ⟶ 27
Arrhythmias: There was 1 episode of second degree AV block during REM sleep. ⟶ 28

MOVEMENT PARAMETERS

	#	Index	
Total periodic leg movements in sleep (PLMS)	0	0.0	per hour of sleep
PLMS resulting in arousal	0	0.0	per hour of sleep
Duration of arousals	-	seconds	
Total nonperiodic leg movements in sleep (NPLMS)	0	0.0	per hour of sleep
NPLMS resulting in arousal	0	0.0	per hour of sleep
Duration of arousals	-	seconds	

ADDITIONAL FINDINGS

The patient reported that she slept much better than usual and awoke feeling much more alert and awake than usual. ⟶ 29

MEDICATIONS

Type	Amount	When taken
None		

FIGURE C5-9
CPAP report, page 2.

MORNING QUESTIONNAIRE

All things considered, your sleep last night was

(circle one answer)

1. Much better than usual
2. Better than usual
3. Same as usual
4. Worse than usual
5. Much worse than usual

Compared to the way you usually feel after awakening do you

1. Feel much more alert and awake than usual
2. Feel more alert and awake than usual
3. Feel same as usual
4. Feel less alert and awake than usual
5. Feel much less alert and wake than usual

How long did it take you to fall asleep last night? _5 mins._

30

Compared to the usual time it takes you to fall asleep, this was
1. Much shorter
2. Shorter
3. Same
4. Longer
5. Much longer

How many hours/minutes did you sleep last night? _5.5 hrs./mins._

Compared to the usual time you sleep at home, this was
1. Much longer
2. Longer
3. Same
4. Shorter
5. Much shorter

How many times did you awaken last night? _1 time_

Compared to the usual number of times your waken, this was
1. Many fewer than usual
2. Fewer than usual
3. Same
4. More than usual
5. Many more than usual

FIGURE C5-10
Post-CPAP morning questionnaire.

FINAL SYNTHESIS

This case is an important example of the balance that should be maintained between a good clinical history and the results of an "objective" diagnostic study. Diagnostic sleep studies are not always the most powerful part of the diagnostic process. Sleep studies can be affected in unpredictable ways, with unusual results that may run counter to initial expectations. Initial diagnostic impressions based on the clinical history should not be abandoned just because the sleep study does not lend support.

Additionally, this case is a dramatic example of the reasons why strict sleep laboratory protocols must be implemented. The addition of a second pillow by the patient—just because it was available in the sleep laboratory and the technologist on duty was accommodating—resulted in a change in sleep and respiratory parameters that could have left the patient improperly diagnosed and therefore untreated.

Case 6

PRESENTING COMPLAINT

"My snoring is ruining my marriage."

PATIENT DEMOGRAPHICS

The patient is a 52-year-old, white male, a sales representative.

PATIENT SLEEP HISTORY

The patient reports snoring for at least six or seven years, with the loudness increasing significantly in the last six months. The patient's wife reports numerous snore-related arousals and movements each night. Additionally, she reports periods of apparent apnea lasting up to 60 sec. The patient is an obligatory mouth breather and often awakens with a headache. The patient complains of nocturia, with three to five trips to the bathroom each night.

The patient typically gets into bed around 1 AM and gets up before 8 AM.

MEDICAL HISTORY AND EXAM

The patient is 5'10" and weighs 265 lbs. He has had a 50 lbs weight gain over the last five years. His medical history is significant for diabetes mellitus and hypertension. Medications are insulin and Capoten 12.5 daily. On examination, the nasopharynx was mildly crowed. The examination otherwise was unremarkable.

PRELIMINARY DIAGNOSIS

A preliminary diagnosis of obstructive sleep apnea was made.

PLAN

A diagnostic polysomnogram (DPSG) was ordered. An MSLT was not scheduled, as diagnoses other than sleep apnea were thought to be unlikely.

COMMENTARY ON CLINICAL MATERIALS

All boxed numbers in the figures refer to the following comments.

Sleep Log (Figure C6-1)

1. A review of the sleep log shows sleep not to be as disrupted as described by the patient during his initial evaluation. Usual bedtimes appear earlier, and few awakenings from sleep are present. It is impossible to determine if the sleep log accurately reflects the patient's perceptions or whether the sleep log was not filled out on a daily basis as instructed. Many patients appear to fill out all seven days/nights of the sleep log at the same time. This practice will result in less detail and less accurate data.

Bedtime Questionnaire (Figure C6-2)

2. Bedtime and wake time, as noted on this questionnaire, are not identical to those noted during the initial evaluation, suggesting that the sleep log data may not be accurate.

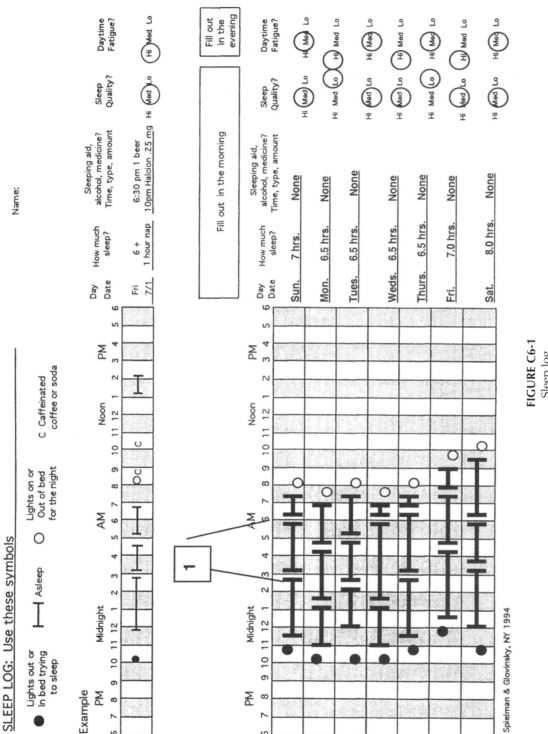

FIGURE C6-1
Sleep log.

BEDTIME QUESTIONNAIRE

How sleepy do you feel right now? Place mark along line.

Very sleepy_____✕_____ Very Alert

Please describe how you feel now. Circle one of the numbers on the Stanford Sleepiness Scale below:

1. Alert. Wide Awake. Energetic.
2. Functioning at a high level, but not at peak. Able to concentrate.
3. Awake, but not fully alert.
4. A little foggy, let down.
5. Foggy. Beginning to lose interest in remaining awake. Slowed down.
6. Cannot stay awake. Sleep onset soon.

Please describe your sleep last night:

What time did you turn out the lights?	1 AM	
How long did it take to fall asleep?	15 mins.	
How many hours/minutes did you sleep last night?	6.5 hrs.	
What time did you awaken this morning?	8 AM	
How many times did you awaken last night?	3	

Did you nap or fall asleep today?   Yes   No
If YES, please indicate at what times and for how long
_____

Was today a typical day?   Yes   No
If NO, please explain
_____

How well do you expect to sleep tonight?
Not very well, I don't sleep well away from home_____

Do you feel ready to go to sleep right now?   Yes   No
If NO, please explain
No, I usually go to be later._____

Did you drink any alcohol today?   Yes   No

If YES, please list what kind, how much and when taken
_____

Did you drink any caffeinated beverages (coffee, tea, colas, etc.) today? YES NO

FIGURE C6-2
Pre-DPSG bedtime questionnaire, page 1.

If YES, please what kind, when taken and how much?
4 diet Cokes, 3 cups coffee in morning

Did you smoke any cigarettes, cigars, pipe, etc. today? YES (NO)

If YES, please what kind, when taken and how much?

Please list all medications you took today. Be sure to include prescriptions medications as well as those you take without a prescription

Name	How Much	Reason	When Taken
Insulin			

Please list any other medication you will be taking before going to sleep

Name	How Much	Reason	When Taken
Unisom			
Benadryl			

3

Please list any other medication you have stopped taking in the last 30 days.

Name	How Much	Reason	When Taken
None			

Please describe anything else that occurred last night or today that might affect your sleep tonight.

FIGURE C6-2
Pre-DPSG bedtime questionnaire, page 2.

3. The patient takes over-the-counter hypnotics, apparently to reduce the number of awakenings from sleep. Use of hypnotic or sedative medications may increase the duration of apneas and hypopneas or interfere with arousal mechanisms that result in the termination of apneas and hypopneas. These medications were not mentioned by the patient during his initial evaluation.

Diagnostic Polysomnogram (Figure C6-3)

4. Sleep parameters show severe sleep fragmentation, with light stage 1 sleep accounting for over 85% of total sleep instead of the 10% or less expected for a patient of this age.

5. Deep sleep was completely absent and REM sleep occurred in quantities less than expected.

6. Sleep fragmentation was characterized by a larger number of longer periods of wakefulness, lasting 1–5 minutes each.

7. Severe obstructive sleep apnea is present, with frequent O_2 desaturations to <50%.

8. Obstructive sleep apnea does not depend on body position but is equally severe in all positions.

9. Periodic leg movements in sleep (PLMS) are not present; but with sleep fragmentation this severe, the appearance of PLMS (a repetitive disorder) may not be possible.

Diagnostic Polysomnogram Histogram (Figure C6-4)

10. REM sleep periods are discernible but severely fragmented.

11. A change to left lateral decubitus position resulted in less severe O_2 desaturations and a change from fully obstructive apneas to primarily hypopneas. However, repetitive episodes of sleep-disordered breathing continued until the end of the recording.

12. The most severe hypoxia is associated with REM sleep.

Morning Questionnaire (Figure C6-5)

The patient estimated total sleep time as 7 hr when less than 4 hr of sleep were present. With such a high level of sleep fragmentation, accurate subjective estimations of sleep are not possible. The estimate of 7 hr appears to reflect total recording time.

Sample Interpretation

This recording is remarkable for the sleep-disordered breathing. A total of 749 obstructive apneas and hypopneas were noted for a respiratory disturbance index (RDI) of 203.3/hr of sleep. All apneas and hypopneas were associated with significant decreases in SaO_2, with <50% the lowest value noted. Apneas and hypopneas typically ranged from 19 to 29.9 sec, with the longest event lasting 47.5 sec. Loud, disruptive snoring was present throughout.

Sleep quality was much poorer than expected. Light, stage 1 sleep accounted for more than 85% of total sleep time instead of the expected 10% or less. Deep sleep was absent and REM sleep occurred in quantities lower than expected. Frequent brief arousals were present but too short to be quantified using the standard conventions of sleep analysis.

In summary, these findings are consistent with severe obstructive sleep apnea.

Note: As the diagnostic polysomnogram was consistent with severe obstructive sleep apnea, the patient returned for a treatment trial of continuous positive airway pressure (CPAP).

Pre-Continuous Positive Airway Pressure Bedtime Questionnaire (Figure C6-6)

13. The patient maintained a late bedtime.

Continuous Positive Airway Pressure Treatment Trial Report (Figure C6-7)

14. Sleep data are divided according to CPAP pressure. Data acquired during each pressure level are presented as if they were the results of "mini" sleep studies. In this way, the effects of different pressures can be compared directly. For instance, it can be seen that significant quantities of REM sleep are present at both the 7.5 and 10.0 cm H_2O pressures.

15. The patient's subjective assessment of the quality of his sleep and AM alertness often is related to the willingness to accept CPAP treatment at home and compliance with treatment.

16. A review of pressure levels show all to be effective when compared to the RDI of 203.3/hr sleep during the diagnostic polysomnogram.

Sleep Parameters
General

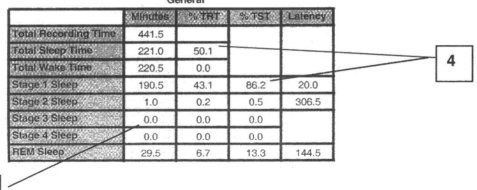

	Minutes	% TRT	% TST	Latency
Total Recording Time	441.5			
Total Sleep Time	221.0	50.1		
Total Wake Time	220.5	0.0		
Stage 1 Sleep	190.5	43.1	86.2	20.0
Stage 2 Sleep	1.0	0.2	0.5	306.5
Stage 3 Sleep	0.0	0.0	0.0	
Stage 4 Sleep	0.0	0.0	0.0	
REM Sleep	29.5	6.7	13.3	144.5

4

5

Sleep Continuity Measures

Sleep Efficiency (%)	50.1
Wake After Sleep Onset (Min)	200.5
# of Awakenings > 5 Minutes	3.0
# of Awakenings > 1 Min & < 5 Min	180.0
# of Arousals (all sources)	749.0
Arousal Index (hr. of sleep)	203.3

6

Patient Sleep Estimations

	Subjective	Objective
Total Recording Time	7	3.7
Total Sleep Time	45	20.0
Total Sleep Time	5	3.0

Patient Evaluation of Laboratory Sleep Compared to Usual Sleep

All in All	Worse than usual
AM Alertness	Feel same as usual

FIGURE C6-3
Polysomnogram (DPSG) report, page 1.

SLEEP DISORDERED BREATHING

	Obstructive Apneas		Hypopneas		Central Apneas		Totals		
	REM	NREM	REM	NREM	REM	NREM	REM	NREM	Total
#	24.0	219.0	21.0	485.0	0.0	0.0	45.0	704.0	749.0
Index	48.8	68.6	42.7	152.5	0.0	0.0	91.5	221.4	203.3
Average Duration	29.9	22.9	19.0	20.1	0.0	0.0			
Maximum Duration	44.9	47.5	33.8	38.4	0.0	0.0			
Average SaO2%	55.0	64.0	76.0	76.0	0.0	0.0			
Low SaO2%	50.0	50.0	60.0	50.0	0.0	0.0			

7

Body Position Effects

	Supine	Prone	Left	Right
Total Recording Time	170.6	0.0	199.8	71.1
Total Sleep Time	74.6	0.0	107.0	39.4
Sleep Efficiency	43.7	0.0	53.5	55.4
RDI	103.7	0.0	106.5	103.6
Low SaO2	50.0	0.0	50.0	50.0

8

Baseline Cardiorespiratory Parameters

	Wake		REM		NREM	
	High	Low	High	Low	High	Low
SaO2 (%)	92.0	91.0	90.0	39.0	83.0	50.0
Respiratory Rate	18.0	16.0	18.0	16.0	18.0	14.0
ECG	91.0	90.0	87.0	67.0	88.0	79.0

Other Cardiorespiratory Data

Snoring	Very loud
Cardiac Arrhythmia	variable sinus rhythm
Undisturbed Sleep (hrs.)	0.0
Paradoxical Movements	During respiratory events

FIGURE C6-3
Polysomnogram (DPSG) report, page 2.

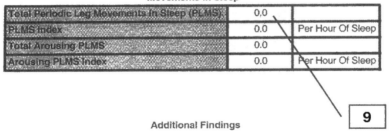

Movements in Sleep

Total Periodic Leg Movements in Sleep (PLMS)	0.0	
PLMS Index	0.0	Per Hour Of Sleep
Total Arousing PLMS	0.0	
Arousing PLMS Index	0.0	Per Hour Of Sleep

9

Additional Findings

None.

Medication	Quantity	Time Taken
Insulin		
Capoten		

FIGURE C6-3
Polysomnogram (DPSG) report, page 3.

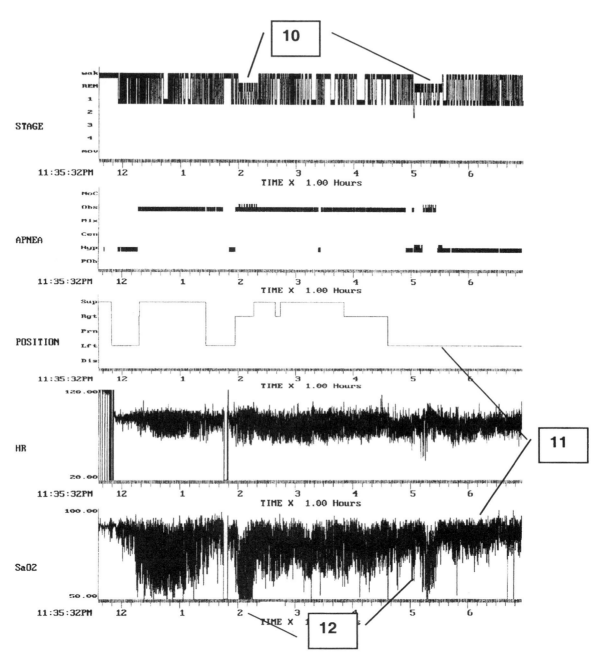

FIGURE C6-4
Polysomnogram (DPSG) histogram.

MORNING QUESTIONNAIRE

All things considered, your sleep last night was

(circle one answer)

1. Much better than usual
2. Better than usual
3. Same as usual
4. Worse than usual
5. Much worse than usual

Compared to the way you usually feel after awakening do you

1. Feel much more alert and awake than usual
2. Feel more alert and awake than usual
3. Feel same as usual
4. Feel less alert and awake than usual
5. Feel much less alert and wake than usual

How long did it take you to fall asleep last night? 45 mins.

Compared to the usual time it takes you to fall asleep, this was
1. Much shorter
2. Shorter
3. Same
4. Longer
5. Much longer

How many hours/minutes did you sleep last night? 7.0 hrs./

Compared to the usual time you sleep at home, this was
1. Much longer
2. Longer
3. Same
4. Shorter
5. Much shorter

How many times did you awaken last night?   5 times

Compared to the usual number of times your waken, this was
1. Many fewer than usual
2. Fewer than usual
3. Same
4. More than usual
5. Many more than usual

FIGURE C6-5
Post-DPSG morning questionnaire.

BEDTIME QUESTIONNAIRE

How sleepy do you feel right now? Place mark along line.

Very sleepy_____✕_____ Very Alert

Please describe how you feel now. Circle one of the numbers on the Stanford Sleepiness Scale below:

1. Alert. Wide Awake. Energetic.
2. Functioning at a high level, but not at peak. Able to concentrate.
3. Awake, but not fully alert.
4. A little foggy, let down.
5. Foggy. Beginning to lose interest in remaining awake. Slowed down.
6. Cannot stay awake. Sleep onset soon.

Please describe your sleep last night:

What time did you turn out the lights?	1:15 AM
How long did it take to fall asleep?	15 mins.
How many hours/minutes did you sleep last night?	5 hrs.
What time did you awaken this morning?	7 AM
How many times did you awaken last night?	2

13

Did you nap or fall asleep today?   Yes   (No)
If YES, please indicate at what times and for how long
_____

Was today a typical day?   (Yes)   No
If NO, please explain
_____

How well do you expect to sleep tonight?
Very well
_____

Do you feel ready to go to sleep right now?   (Yes)   No
If NO, please explain
_____

Did you drink any alcohol today?   (Yes)   No

If YES, please list what kind, how much and when taken
2 glasses wine at dinner 6 PM
_____

Did you drink any caffeinated beverages (coffee, tea, colas, etc.) today? (YES) NO

FIGURE C6-6
Pre-CPAP bedtime questionnaire, page 1.

If YES, please what kind, when taken and how much?
1 cup coffee at breakfast
_____

Did you smoke any cigarettes, cigars, pipe, etc. today?   YES (NO)

If YES, please what kind, when taken and how much?

_____

Please list all medications you took today. Be sure to include prescriptions
medications as well as those you take without a prescription

Name	How Much	Reason	When Taken
Insulin	____	____	____
____	____	____	____
____	____	____	____
____	____	____	____
____	____	____	____
____	____	____	____
____	____	____	____
____	____	____	____

Please list any other medication you will be taking before going to sleep

Name	How Much	Reason	When Taken
Unisom	____	____	____
____	____	____	____
____	____	____	____
____	____	____	____
____	____	____	____

Please list any other medication you have stopped taking in the last 30 days.

Name	How Much	Reason	When Taken
None	____	____	____
____	____	____	____
____	____	____	____

Please describe anything else that occurred last night or today that might affect
your sleep tonight.
_____

FIGURE C6-6
Pre-CPAP bedtime questionnaire, page 2.

Lights Out	11:28:24PM	On	6:13:24AM

Sleep Parameters
General

Total Recording Time	405.0
Total Sleep Time	378.0

SLEEP PARAMETERS BY PRESSURE LEVEL

NCPAP Pressures (cm H2O)			
	5	7.5	10
Total Recording Time	91.8	224.9	88.3
Total Sleep Time	80.5	210.7	86.8
Wake Time (mins)	11.3	14.2	1.5
Sleep Efficiency (%)	87.7	93.7	98.3
Stage 1 Sleep (min)	7.0	7.5	3.0
Stage 1 Sleep (%)	8.7	3.6	3.5
Stage 2 Sleep (min)	9.0	98.2	18.3
Stage 2 Sleep (%)	11.2	46.6	21.1
Stage 3 Sleep (min)	9.0	31.0	0.0
Stage 3 Sleep (%)	11.2	14.7	0.0
Stage 4 Sleep (min)	17.0	10.5	0.0
Stage 4 Sleep (%)	21.1	5.0	0.0
REM Sleep (mins)	38.5	63.5	65.5
REM Sleep (%)	47.8	30.1	75.5
Arousal Index (per hr.)	32.0	3.1	2.8

14

Patient Sleep Estimations

	Subjective	Objective
Total Recording Time	6.5	6.3
Total Sleep Time	===	10.5
Total Sleep Time	3	1.0

15

Patient Evaluation of Laboratory Sleep Compared to Usual Sleep

All in All	Better than usual
AM Alertness	Feel same as usual

FIGURE C6-7
CPAP report, page 1.

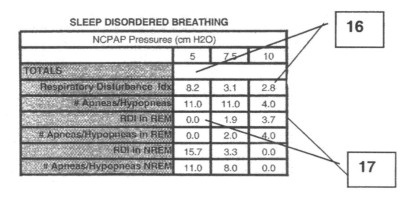

SLEEP DISORDERED BREATHING

NCPAP Pressures (cm H2O)			
	5	7.5	10
TOTALS			
Respiratory Disturbance Idx	8.2	3.1	2.8
# Apneas/Hypopneas	11.0	11.0	4.0
RDI in REM	0.0	1.9	3.7
# Apneas/Hypopneas in REM	0.0	2.0	4.0
RDI in NREM	15.7	3.3	0.0
# Apneas/Hypopneas NREM	11.0	8.0	0.0

16

17

OBSTRUCTIVE APNEA

TOTALS			
# Obstructive Sleep Apneas	0.0	1.0	0.0
Index (hr. of sleep)	0	0	0
REM Sleep			
# Apneas	0.0	0.0	0.0
Index (per hr.)	0.0	0.0	0.0
Average Duration	0.0	0.0	0.0
Maximum Duration	0.0	0.0	0.0
Average SaO2%	0.0	0.0	0.0
Low SaO2%	0.0	0.0	0.0
NREM Sleep			
# Apneas	0.0	0.0	0.0
Index (per hr.)	0.0	0.0	0.0
Average Duration	0.0	0.0	0.0
Maximum Duration	0.0	0.0	0.0
Average SaO2%	0.0	0.0	0.0
Low SaO2%	0.0	0.0	0.0

FIGURE C6-7
CPAP report, page 2.

NCPAP Pressures (cm H2O)			
	5	7.5	10
HYPOPNEAS			
TOTALS			
# of Hypopneas	11.0	10.0	4.0
Index (hr. of sleep)	15.7	5.2	3.7
REM Sleep			
# Hypopneas	0.0	2.0	4.0
Index (per hr.)	0.0	1.9	3.7
Average Duration	0.0	16.4	17.1
Maximum Duration	0.0	17.8	19.9
Average SaO2%	0.0	90.0	91.0
Low SaO2%	0.0	89.0	90.0
NREM Sleep			
# Hypopneas	11.0	8.0	0.0
Index (per hr.)	15.7	3.3	0.0
Average Duration	16.2	16.4	0.0
Maximum Duration	24.8	18.0	0.0
Average SaO2%	86.0	89.0	0.0
Low SaO2%	79.0	83.0	0.0

18

CENTRAL APNEA			
TOTALS			
# Central Sleep Apneas	0.0	0.0	0.0
Index (hr. of sleep)	0	0	0
REM Sleep			
# Central Apneas	0.0	0.0	0.0
Index (per hr.)	0.0	0.0	0.0
Average Duration	0.0	0.0	0.0
Maximum Duration	0.0	0.0	0.0
Average SaO2%	0.0	0.0	0.0
Low SaO2%	0.0	0.0	0.0
NREM Sleep			
# Central Apneas	0.0	0.0	0.0
Index (per hr.)	0.0	0.0	0.0
Average Duration	0.0	0.0	0.0
Maximum Duration	0.0	0.0	0.0
Average SaO2%	0.0	0.0	0.0
Low SaO2%	0.0	0.0	0.0

FIGURE C6-7
CPAP report, page 3.

BODY POSITION EFFECTS

NCPAP Pressures (cm H2O)			
	5	7.5	10
Total Recording Time - Supine	0.1	225.0	88.3
Total Recording Time - Prone	0.0	0.0	0.0
Total Recording Time - Left	91.9	0.0	0.0
Total Recording Time - Right	0.0	0.0	0.0
Total Sleep Time - Supine	0.0	210.7	86.8
Total Sleep Time - Prone	0.0	0.0	0.0
Total Sleep Time - Left	80.5	0.0	0.0
Total Sleep Time - Right	0.0	0.0	0.0
Sleep Efficiency - Supine	0.0	93.7	98.3
Sleep Efficiency - Prone	0.0	0.0	0.0
Sleep Efficiency - Left	87.6	0.0	0.0
Sleep Efficiency - Right	0.0	0.0	0.0
Total RDI - Supine	0.0	2.0	2.8
Total RDI - Prone	0.0	0.0	0.0
Total RDI - Left	5.2	0.0	0.0
Total RDI - Right	0.0	0.0	0.0

Baseline Cardiorespiratory Parameters

	Wake		REM		NREM	
	High	Low	High	Low	High	Low
SaO2 (%)	98.0	95.0	95.0	90.0	95.0	91.0
Respiratory Rate	17.0	14.0	27.0	15.0	18.0	14.0
ECG	97.0	73.0	111.0	66.0	91.0	68.0

Other Cardiorespiratory Data   [19]

Snoring	Eliminated with 10 cm H2O.
Cardiac Arrhythmia	None.
Undisturbed Sleep (hrs.)	5.5
Paradoxical Movements	During respiratory events

Movements in Sleep   [20]

Total Periodic Leg Movements in Sleep (PLMS)	51.0	
PLMS Index	8.1	Per Hour Of Sleep
Total Arousing PLMS	32.0	
Arousing PLMS Index	5.1	Per Hour Of Sleep

FIGURE C6-7
CPAP report, page 4.

Additional Findings

None.

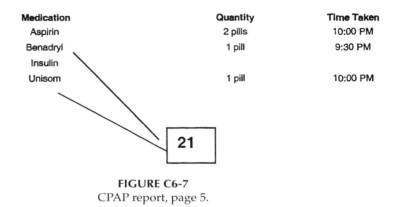

FIGURE C6-7
CPAP report, page 5.

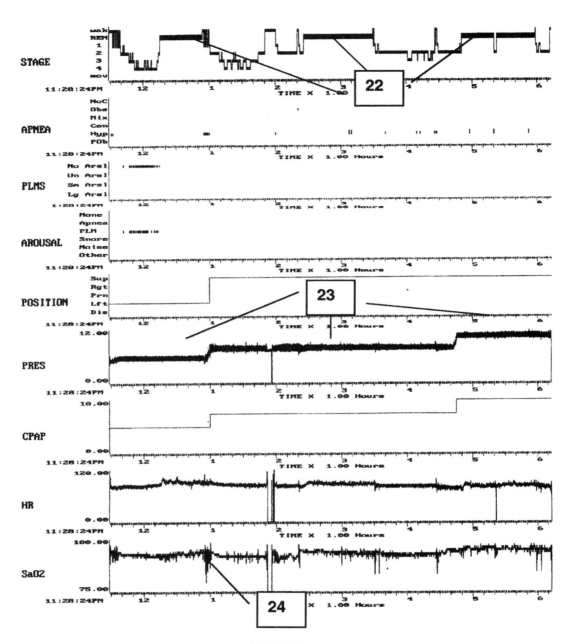

FIGURE C6-8
CPAP histogram.

MORNING QUESTIONNAIRE

All things considered, your sleep last night was

(circle one answer)

1. Much better than usual
2. Better than usual
3. Same as usual
4. Worse than usual
5. Much worse than usual

25 Compared to the way you usually feel after awakening do you

1. Feel much more alert and awake than usual
2. Feel more alert and awake than usual
3. Feel same as usual
4. Feel less alert and awake than usual
5. Feel much less alert and wake than usual

How long did it take you to fall asleep last night? _0 mins._

Compared to the usual time it takes you to fall asleep, this was
1. Much shorter
2. Shorter
3. Same
4. Longer
5. Much longer

How many hours/minutes did you sleep last night? _6.5 hrs./mins._

Compared to the usual time you sleep at home, this was
1. Much longer
2. Longer
3. Same
4. Shorter
5. Much shorter

How many times did you awaken last night? _3 times_

Compared to the usual number of times your waken, this was
1. Many fewer than usual
2. Fewer than usual
3. Same
4. More than usual
5. Many more than usual

FIGURE C6-9
Post-CPAP morning questionnaire.

17. The effectiveness of a particular pressure level can be properly determined only if it was applied when exacerbating factors, such as supine position and REM sleep, were present. In this case, pressures of 7.5 and 10 cm H_2O were administered with the patient in the supine position and during REM sleep.

18. Respiratory data also may be broken down among different types of sleep-disordered breathing. Lower levels of CPAP may result in a change from fully obstructive apneas to hypopneas and higher levels from hypopneas to snoring.

19. Successful CPAP treatment should include maximum reduction in all types of sleep-disordered breathing, including snoring.

20. With the elimination of sleep-disordered breathing, other sleep disorders, such as periodic leg movements in sleep, may be manifested and become a source of sleep fragmentation that require treatment.

21. When patients insist on continuing to use over-the-counter sedatives that might affect the severity of sleep-disordered breathing, the patient should take this medication on the CPAP titration night.

Continuous Positive Airway Pressure Treatment Trial Histogram (Figure C6-8)

22. The CPAP histogram shows sleep architecture as resulting in both deep sleep and REM sleep rebound.

23. Pressure tracing shows increase in CPAP pressures across the recording.

24. At the initial CPAP pressure administered, REM-sleep-related hypoxia persists, resulting in a further increase in pressure.

Sample Interpretation

Administration of a CPAP pressure of 7.5 cm H_2O resulted in a change in the respiratory distur-bance index (RDI) from 203.3/hr of sleep, as noted in the prior diagnostic sleep study, to an RDI of 3.1/hr of sleep. Snoring also was eliminated at this pressure level.

The quality of sleep showed significant improvement with administration of CPAP. Light, stage 1 sleep decreased, while deep sleep and REM sleep increased significantly. The high quantity and percentage of REM sleep and deep sleep (stages 3 and 4) suggests the presence of rebound sleep. Sleep-disordered breathing often results in arousal during sleep, causing a significant reduction or elimination of both deep sleep and REM sleep. When obstructive apneas and hypopneas are eliminated by CPAP, the associated arousals also are eliminated. This often results in an increase in deep sleep and REM sleep well above expected quantities and percentages. Rebound sleep generally is considered an excellent sign of successful treatment. The patient reported sleeping better than usual.

In summary, administration of CPAP at a pressure of 7.5 cm H_2O resulted in a significant reduction in sleep-disordered breathing as well as improvement in sleep quality and daytime alertness.

Morning Questionnaire (Figure C6-9)

25. The significant improvement in objective sleep and respiratory parameters is reflected in the patient subjective estimation of sleep quantity and quality.

FINAL SYNTHESIS

The materials presented here describe a typical case of severe obstructive sleep apnea with successful CPAP treatment.

Case 7

PRESENTING COMPLAINT

"I wake up ten times a night and I am very tired during the day."

PATIENT DEMOGRAPHICS

The patient is a 34-year-old, African-American male, married, research technician.

PATIENT SLEEP HISTORY

The patient has an 18-year history of excessive daytime sleepiness. He has fallen asleep during classes, both in high school and college. Currently, he experiences sleepiness most often while driving but has had no car accidents. He also becomes very sleepy or falls asleep in any situation during which he is physically inactive. He has dozed during conversations, at work while using a computer, while watching TV or movies, and often while reading. The patient reports that he often awakens feeling unrefreshed or groggy and his sleepiness is much worse in the morning and early afternoon but persists at a lower level later in the day. During the workweek he may take one or two unplanned naps per day, lasting 1–10 min each. On weekends, he additionally takes a planned 1 hr nap in midafternoon. The patient does not always find naps refreshing. However, he often recalls a vivid dream during naps.

During the workweek, he reports getting into bed between 11 and 11:30 PM and awakens between 7:30 and 8:00 AM, for a total sleep time of 6.5–8.5 hr. On weekends, he goes to sleep between 1 and 2 AM and often sleeps until 11 AM or noon, for a total sleep time of 9–11 hr. The patient reports 3–10 awakenings per night, each lasting approximately 10 min. He reports that about 20% of all awakenings are associated with gasping or choking and 50% or more are associated with dreaming. On two occasions in the last year, he fell out of bed during a dream. He also reports his mouth to be quite dry upon awakening from sleep.

The patient has no history consistent with cataplexy, sleep paralysis, or hypnogogic hallucination. There is no family history of daytime sleepiness or any other sleep disorder.

The patient is not reported to snore. However, as noted, he awakens almost nightly gasping for breathing and with a dry mouth, suggesting mouth breathing. During the day he has no difficulty with nasal breathing and does not complain of nasal congestion.

MEDICAL HISTORY AND EXAM

On examination the patient is 5'9" and weighs 176 lbs. His blood pressure was 110/70 and pulse was 62 and regular. ENT and neurological exams were normal. Patient has never been hospitalized. Patient does not smoke and is taking no prescription or over-the-counter (OTC) medication. Patient drinks three 16 oz cans of cola each day but no coffee. On interview, the patient had no signs or symptoms of anxiety, depression, or other psychological disorder.

PRELIMINARY DIAGNOSES

1. Narcolepsy:
   Pro—Onset of daytime sleepiness in early teens, reports of vivid dreaming during naps.
   Con—No auxiliary symptoms of narcolepsy, such as cataplexy or sleep paralysis.
2. Obstructive sleep apnea:
   Pro—Gasping arousals from sleep, unrefreshing sleep, AM dry mouth.
3. Insufficient sleep:
   Pro—May sleep 10–12 hr on weekend nights.
4. Nightmares or night terrors.

PLAN

1. Diagnostic polysomnogram (DPSG).
2. Multiple Sleep Latency Test (MSLT).

COMMENTARY ON CLINICAL MATERIALS

All boxed numbers in the figures refer to the following comments.

Sleep Log (Figure C7-1)

1. The sleep log shows frequent awakenings from sleep, consistent with the patient's presenting complaints.
2. Longer naps are present during weekend days, with three or four shorter naps present most days recorded.

Bedtime Questionnaire (Figure C7-2)

3. Questionnaire confirms typical pattern of sleep with frequent awakenings and four to six brief naps during the daytime.

Diagnostic Polysomnogram (Figures C7-3 and C7-4)

4. Slightly more than 6 hr of sleep were recorded, close enough to his reported sleep times to provide hope of a typical night of sleep.
5. Rapid eye movement (REM) sleep quantity and percentage are at the high end of normal for a patient of this age.
6. An overall respiratory disturbance index (RDI) of 19.7/hr was present, but episodes of sleep-disor-

dered breathing occurred much more frequently during REM sleep. Apneas and hypopneas were associated with minor O_2 desaturation, with 91% the lowest SaO_2 value of the entire recording. Therefore, REM sleep fragmentation is the major consequence of these apneas and hypopneas.

7. The REM-sleep-related episodes of sleep-disordered breathing were not characterized by the frequent changes in respiratory rate and amplitude that are part of the normal physiology of REM sleep. Rather, crescendo patterns of snoring with loud terminating snores and snorts were present.
8. The association of sleep-disordered breathing with REM sleep easily is seen without summary data by working downward through the stacked histograms.

Morning Questionnaire (Figure C7-5)

9. The patient reports sleeping better in the sleep laboratory than his home bedroom. This may simply reflect the fact that sleep laboratory rooms often are darker and quieter than home bedrooms.

Sample Interpretation

This recording is remarkable for the sleep-disordered breathing. A total of 124 apneas and hypopneas were recorded, for an overall respiratory disturbance index of 19.7/hr of sleep. Apneas and hypopneas occurred more frequently during REM sleep, for a REM sleep index of 42.5/hr of sleep. Apneas and hypopneas generally were short in duration, with the maximum duration noted at 33 sec. Apneas and hypopneas were associated with 3–5% O_2 desaturation, with the maximum O_2 desaturation to 91%. Snoring was noted throughout the recording. ECG was unremarkable.

The overall quality and quantity of sleep was surprisingly good, in light of the frequent apneas and hypopneas. Light, stage 1 sleep was only slightly elevated, and good quantities of deep sleep and REM sleep were noted. REM sleep, however, was severely fragmented by apneas and hypopneas. Apneas and hypopneas were associated with frequent, but brief, arousals that did not always result in a change in sleep stage. Due to their briefness and the fact that the standard conventions of sleep staging permit no quantification of arousals lasting less than 15 sec, these arousals

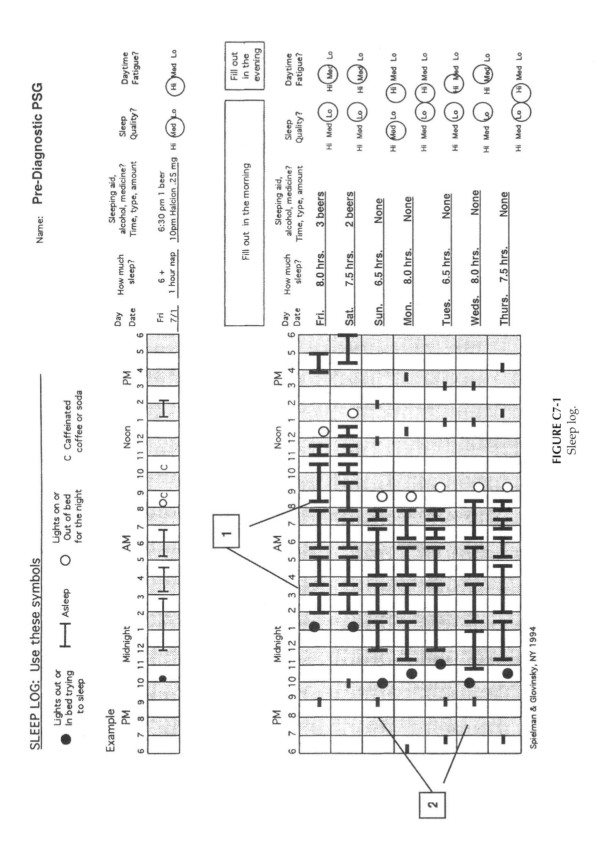

FIGURE C7-1
Sleep log.

BEDTIME QUESTIONNAIRE

How sleepy do you feel right now? Place mark along line.

Very sleepy_____✕_____ Very Alert

Please describe how you feel now. Circle one of the numbers on the Stanford Sleepiness Scale below:

1. Alert. Wide Awake. Energetic.
2. Functioning at a high level, but not at peak. Able to concentrate.
3. Awake, but not fully alert.
4. A little foggy, let down.
5. Foggy. Beginning to lose interest in remaining awake. Slowed down.
6. Cannot stay awake. Sleep onset soon.

Please describe your sleep last night:

What time did you turn out the lights?	11:00 PM
How long did it take to fall asleep?	60?
How many hours/minutes did you sleep last night?	6.5 hrs.
What time did you awaken this morning?	6:15 AM
How many times did you awaken last night?	5-10 3

Did you nap or fall asleep today?   Yes   No
If YES, please indicate at what times and for how long 2-3 times in AM for 1-2 mins. and 1-2 times in afternoon for about 5 minutes.

Was today a typical day?   Yes   No
If NO, please explain

How well do you expect to sleep tonight?
Not well, I never do.

Do you feel ready to go to sleep right now?   Yes   No
If NO, please explain
I feel too awake.

Did you drink any alcohol today?   Yes   No

If YES, please list what kind, how much and when taken

Did you drink any caffeinated beverages (coffee, tea, colas, etc.) today? YES NO

FIGURE C7-2
Pre-DPSG bedtime questionnaire, page 1.

If YES, please what kind, when taken and how much?
3 colas last one at 3 PM
_____

Did you smoke any cigarettes, cigars, pipe, etc. today?   YES NO

If YES, please what kind, when taken and how much?

_____

Please list all medications you took today. Be sure to include prescriptions medications as well as those you take without a prescription

Name	How Much	Reason	When Taken
None.			

Please list any other medication you will be taking before going to sleep

Name	How Much	Reason	When Taken
None			

Please list any other medication you have stopped taking in the last 30 days.

Name	How Much	Reason	When Taken
None			

Please describe anything else that occurred last night or today that might affect your sleep tonight. _____
_____

FIGURE C7-2
Pre-DPSG bedtime questionnaire, page 2.

POLYSOMNOGRAM REPORT

Lights off: 11:28 PM   Lights on: 6:51 AM

SLEEP PARAMETERS

GENERAL		
Total Time in Bed	418.0	mins.
Total Sleep Time	**377.5**	mins.
Total Wake Time	40.5	mins.
Sleep Efficiency	**85.4**	%
	4	

SLEEP STAGING				
Stage 1	30.0	min	7.9	%
Stage 2	165.0	min	43.7	%
Stage 3	18.0	min	4.8	%
Stage 4	51.5	min	13.6	%
REM	113.0	min	29.9	%
			5	

LATENCIES		
Latency to stage 1	**17.0**	mins.
Latency to stage 2	13.5	mins.
Latency to REM	**77.5**	mins.

WAKETIME		
Wake between sleep onset and sleep	21	mins.
Wake after sleep offset	12.5	mins.
Awakenings lasting 1-5 mins.	1	
Awakenings > 5 mins.	1	

SLEEP DISORDERED BREATHING

	Obstructive		Hypopnea		Central		Totals		
	REM	NREM	REM	NREM	REM	NREM	REM	NREM	All
# of apneas/hypopneas	0	0	76	41	4	3	80	44	124
Index (#/hr. of sleep)	-	-	40.0	9.3	2.1	0.68	42.5	10	19.7
Max. Duration (secs)			33	29	26	24			
Avg. Duration (secs.)			22	22	21	20			
Low SaO2 (%)			97	97	95	95			
Avg. SaO2 (%)			96	95	91	93	**6**		
Avg. Arousal (secs.)			6	11	10	9			

BASELINE CARDIORESPIRATORY DATA

	Wake		REM		NREM	
ECG	63-79		57-78		63-75	
Respiratory Rate	14-16		10-18		12-14	
SaO2*	96-99	%	97-98	%	95-96	%

FIGURE C7-3
Polysomnogram (DPSG) report, page 1.

OTHER CARDIORESPIRATORY DATA

Body Position: The patient slept in the prone, supine and right lateral decubitus positions.

Undisturbed sleep: 4 hours.

7

Snoring: Soft to moderately loud snoring was noted during the recording, with the loudest snores and snorts occurring at the termination of apneas and hypopneas and in the supine position.

Arrhythmias: No cardiac arrhythmias noted.

MOVEMENT PARAMETERS

	#	Index	
Total periodic leg movements in sleep (PLMS)	22	3.5	per hour of sleep
PLMS resulting in arousal	18	2.9	per hour of sleep
Duration of arousals	3-6	seconds	
Total nonperiodic leg movements in sleep (NPLMS)	0	0.0	per hour of sleep
NPLMS resulting in arousal	0	0.0	per hour of sleep
Duration of arousals	0	seconds	

ADDITIONAL FINDINGS

None.

MEDICATIONS

Type	Amount	When taken

None noted by patient.

FIGURE C7-3
Polysomnogram (DPSG) report, page 2.

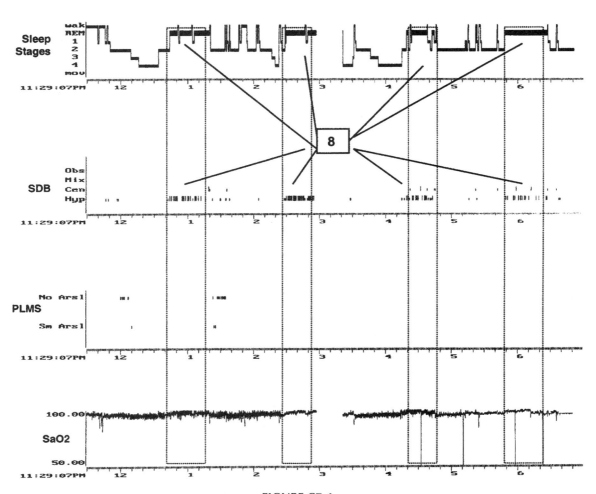

FIGURE C7-4
Polysomnogram (DPSG) histogram.

MORNING QUESTIONNAIRE

All things considered, your sleep last night was

(circle one answer)

    1. Much better than usual
    2. Better than usual
    3. Same as usual
    4. Worse than usual
    5. Much worse than usual

            9

Compared to the way you usually feel after awakening do you

    1. Feel much more alert and awake than usual
    2. Feel more alert and awake than usual
    3. Feel same as usual
    4. Feel less alert and awake than usual
    5. Feel much less alert and wake than usual

How long did it take you to fall asleep last night? <u>30</u> mins.
Compared to the usual time it takes you to fall asleep, this was
    1. Much shorter
    2. Shorter
    3. Same
    4. Longer
    5. Much longer

How many hours/minutes did you sleep last night? <u>6-7</u> hrs./mins.
Compared to the usual time you sleep at home, this was
    1. Much longer
    2. Longer
    3. Same
    4. Shorter
    5. Much shorter

How many times did you awaken last night? <u>4-6</u> times
Compared to the usual number of times your waken, this was
    1. Many fewer than usual
    2. Fewer than usual
    3. Same
    4. More than usual
    5. Many more than usual

FIGURE C7-5
Post-DPSG morning questionnaire, page 1.

Please comment specifically on how your night in the sleep laboratory was different than sleep at home

	Circle one	Describe
Room Temperature	Better (Same) Worse	_____
Mattress	Better Same (Worse)	_____
Pillow	Better Same (Worse)	_____
Noise	Better Same (Worse)	_____
Light	Better (Same) Worse	_____
Sleeping Position	Better (Same) Worse	_____
Blankets	Better (Same) Worse	_____
Sense of Security	Better (Same) Worse	_____
Snacks	Better (Same) Worse	_____
TV	Better (Same) Worse	_____
_____	Better Same Worse	_____
_____	Better Same Worse	_____

In what way was your sleep or the sleeping environment better here than your bedroom at home? __Not_____

In what way was your sleep or the sleeping environment worse here than your bedroom at home? Other patients talking too loud._____

Did anything happen in the sleep laboratory (other than electrodes etc.) that does not usually happen at home? Harder to sleep on stomach._____

Does anything usually happen at home during sleep that did not happen here?
_____

How was the sleep test different from what you expected? _____

_____

Any comments or suggestions? Wireless transmitter??

_____

FIGURE C7-5
Post-DPSG morning questionnaire, page 2.

are not represented in the sleep parameters summary.

In summary, these findings are consistent with a diagnosis of primarily moderate REM-sleep-related obstructive sleep apnea.

Multiple Sleep Latency Test (Figure C7-6)

10. A mean sleep latency of 1.5 min is well within that range of severe daytime sleepiness. Could a very short mean sleep latency of 1.5 min be secondary to a single night with slightly less sleep time than the patient usually reports? Reduction in total sleep time the night before MSLT testing has been reported to result in shorter sleep latencies. What would be the effect of cumulative partial sleep deprivation? It is almost impossible to make an evidence-based decision whether this short mean sleep latency is the result of sleep deprivation, sleep fragmentation from the sleep apnea, or due to narcolepsy.

11. Unambiguous REM sleep was present on the first four nap opportunities. As previously noted, sleep-onset REM periods (SOREMPs) can appear in the MSLT of apparently normal individuals as well as in patients with sleep apnea and other disorders. In this case, the question must be, what is the likelihood that a patient without narcolepsy could have four SOREMPS on an MSLT? Based on current research, the diagnosis of narcolepsy would be most consistent with these findings. However, 10 years ago, the presence of two SOREMPs would have been taken as powerful evidence for the diagnosis of narcolepsy. An additional issue is whether high levels of REM sleep fragmentation caused by sleep-disordered breathing could have potentiated REM sleep sufficiently to produce four SOREMPs.

Sample Interpretation

A mean sleep latency of 1.5 min (to stage 1 sleep) is consistent with the finding of severe daytime sleepiness. The presence of REM sleep in four of the five naps is most consistent with a diagnosis of narcolepsy. However, due to the severe fragmentation of REM sleep by apneas and hypopneas during the prior night's sleep, it is possible that these sleep-onset REM periods resulted from REM sleep deprivation and subsequent rebound.

SYNTHESIS OF DIAGNOSTIC TESTING

The MSLT demonstrated severe daytime sleepiness with four SOREMPs. Under most circumstances, this would be powerful evidence for the diagnosis of narcolepsy. However, the prior night's DPSG demonstrated significant fragmentation of REM sleep (42.0/hr of REM sleep), with the remainder of sleep relatively undisturbed. The high level of REM sleep fragmentation suggests the possibility of persistent, nightly REM sleep deprivation with associated increase in "pressure" for REM sleep that might result in the abnormal appearance of REM sleep on the MSLT.

Additionally, significant sleep apnea was present and appears to be the source of the frequent awakenings from sleep reported by the patient. This is consistent with the patient's reports of awakening gasping for breath and the pattern of awakenings noted on the sleep log, which suggests awakenings occurring with 90–120 min intervals associated with the REM/non-REM cycle.

For these reasons, an unequivocal diagnosis of narcolepsy could not be made at this point. The possible significance of sleep apnea in fragmenting the patient's sleep, depriving the patient of REM sleep and causing the patient's daytime sleepiness, needed to be explored. For this reason, options for treating sleep apnea were reviewed with the patient. As the treatment of sleep apnea essentially is an empirical test of our theory that sleep apnea might be the primary sleep disorder, the patient opted for the least invasive and most easily reversible treatment, nasal continuous positive airway pressure (NCPAP).

If NCPAP is objectively successful in reducing the overall respiratory disturbance index (RDI) and significantly reduces the fragmentation of REM sleep, as can be seen in a REM sleep RDI, the patient will be prescribed the NCPAP for home use and followed for three to four weeks. If the patient reports improvement in daytime alertness and remission of other symptoms, this treatment will continue with no further testing. If, however, the patient reports no significant improvement, the patient will return to the sleep laboratory for a repeat sleep study with administration of NCPAP at the previously determined optimal level for the entire night to be followed by an MSLT. This will allow for alertness testing without the influence of prior sleep apnea.

MULTIPLE SLEEP LATENCY TEST (MSLT) REPORT

DESCRIPTION OF PROCEDURES: The MSLT consists of 5 twenty minute nap opportunities given at 2 hour intervals throughout the course of one day. Patients are instructed to fall asleep as quickly as possible. If sleep occurs the nap is terminated 15 minutes after sleep onset. Patients are not permitted to sleep between scheduled naps. All data are visually scored and analyzed according to standard criteria.

TEST RESULTS

10

LATENCIES (in minutes)						
	10:00 AM	12:00 PM	2:00 PM	4:00 PM	6:00 PM	Mean
First signs of drowsiness	0.0	0.5	0.0	0.5	3.0	0.8
Latency to Stage 1	0.0	3.0	0.5	0.5	3.0	1.5
Latency to Stage 2	15.5	6.5	18.5	10.5	12.0	12.6
Latency to REM	5.5	7.0	1.5	1.5	-	

* A latency of 20 minutes indicates that no sleep occurred in the allotted time.

MEDICATIONS: None

ADDITIONAL DATA: The patient reported that he was as alert as usual during the day.

11

FIGURE C7-6
MSLT report.

COMMENTARY ON CLINICAL MATERIALS FOR THE NASAL CONTINUOUS POSITIVE AIRWAY PRESSURE TREATMENT TRIAL

Again, all boxed numbers refer to the following comments.

Sleep Log

A sleep log was not required prior to performance of the NCPAP treatment trial. However, the patient was requested to keep his usual sleep/wake schedule.

Bedtime Questionnaire (Figure C7-7)

The prior night's sleep does not appear as disrupted as previously noted and the patient did not report any daytime naps.

Nasal Continuous Positive Airway Pressure Treatment Trial (Figure C7-8)

12. With administration of CPAP, REM sleep decreased to the lower range of normal for the patient's age. Deep sleep, however, remained essentially unchanged.
13. Total sleep time was similar to the diagnostic sleep study, although sleep efficiency improved.
14. The RDI was reduced from 19.7/hr of sleep to 2.3/hr of sleep with CPAP.
15. The number and disruptiveness of periodic leg movements increased with CPAP administration, a not uncommon result of successful CPAP administration. Additionally, the patient reported no improvement in his subjective estimation of overall sleep and AM alertness.

Nasal Continuous Positive Airway Pressure Treatment Trial Histogram (Figure C7-9)

16. The histogram demonstrates that residual sleep-disordered breathing is scattered.

Sample Interpretation

Administration of a pressure of 7.5 cm H_2O resulted in a change from a respiratory disturbance index of 19.7/hr of sleep, as recorded during the prior diagnostic sleep study, to an RDI of 2.3/hr of sleep, in this recording. The REM sleep RDI of 42.1/hr of sleep, as noted in the previous sleep study, was reduced to 3.3/hr of REM sleep. This is consistent with a change from moderate obstructive sleep apnea to normal respiration in sleep. Snoring and paradoxical out-of-phase movements of the chest and abdomen noted in the baseline recording also were eliminated at this pressure level.

The quality of sleep showed significant improvement with the administration of NCPAP. The frequent, brief apnea- and hypopnea-related arousals from sleep that characterized the baseline sleep study were essentially eliminated. The patient reported, on the AM questionnaire, sleeping the same as usual.

In summary, the administration of a pressure of 7.5 cm H_2O resulted in change from moderate obstructive sleep apnea to normal respiration in sleep.

SYNTHESIS TO DATE

The patient's comment on his AM questionnaire is not uncommon on the first night of NCPAP treatment and may represent:

1. Difficulty in adapting to the NCPAP apparatus and sensation of positive pressure.
2. Early pressure levels administered did not result in sufficient reduction in sleep-disordered breathing and, therefore, a relatively low quantity of good quality sleep.
3. Sleep apnea is not the source of this patient's daytime sleepiness or, at best, is a minor contributing factor.

An MSLT was not performed immediately following the NCPAP treatment trial because of the many potential difficulties inherent in interpreting the results:

1. An acceptable level of treatment, with reduction in sleep-disordered breathing to normal or near normal levels and improvement in sleep quality while maintaining an acceptable quantity of sleep, often is not possible. The greater the number of NCPAP pressure levels administered, the less likely the patient will awaken in the morning with a "normal" or improved level of alertness.
2. The patient may experience discomfort from the use of the nasal mask and sensation of positive pressure that, in and of themselves, may be a source of sleep fragmentation.

BEDTIME QUESTIONNAIRE (NCPAP)

How sleepy do you feel right now? Place mark along line.

Very sleepy_____✕_____ Very Alert

Please describe how you feel now. Circle one of the numbers on the Stanford Sleepiness Scale below:

1. Alert. Wide Awake. Energetic.
2. Functioning at a high level, but not at peak. Able to concentrate.
3. Awake, but not fully alert.
4. A little foggy, let down.
5. Foggy. Beginning to lose interest in remaining awake. Slowed down.
6. Cannot stay awake. Sleep onset soon.

Please describe your sleep last night:

What time did you turn out the lights?	11:30 PM
How long did it take to fall asleep?	20 minutes
How many hours/minutes did you sleep last night?	6-8 hrs.
What time did you awaken this morning?	6:30 AM
How many times did you awaken last night?	2

Did you nap or fall asleep today?   Yes   (No)
If YES, please indicate at what times and for how long
_____

Was today a typical day?   (Yes)   No
If NO, please explain

How well do you expect to sleep tonight?
? _____

Do you feel ready to go to sleep right now?   Yes   (No)
If NO, please explain

Did you drink any alcohol today?   Yes   (No)

If YES, please list what kind, how much and when taken

FIGURE C7-7
Pre-CPAP bedtime questionnaire, page 1.

Did you drink any caffeinated beverages (coffee, tea, colas, etc.) today? YES NO

If YES, please what kind, when taken and how much?
Cola 18 oz. in PM
_____

Did you smoke any cigarettes, cigars, pipe, etc. today?   YES NO

If YES, please what kind, when taken and how much?
_____

Please list all medications you took today. Be sure to include prescriptions medications as well as those you take without a prescription

Name	How Much	Reason	When Taken
None			

Please list any other medication you will be taking before going to sleep

Name	How Much	Reason	When Taken
None			

Please list any other medication you have stopped taking in the last 30 days.

Name	How Much	Reason	When Taken
None			

Please describe anything else that occurred last night or today that might affect your sleep tonight. _____
_____

FIGURE C7-7
Pre-CPAP bedtime questionnaire, page 2.

Lights out: 12:08 AM   Lights on: 6:15 AM   **12**

SLEEP PARAMETERS

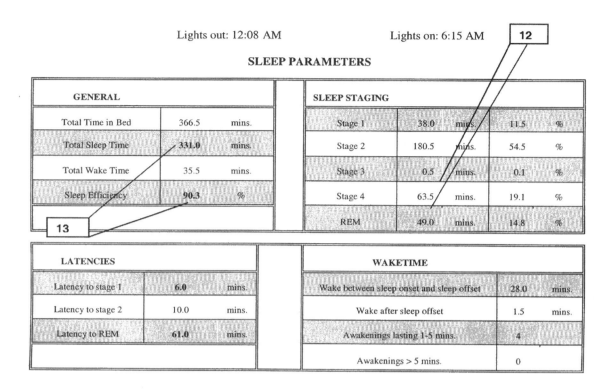

GENERAL		
Total Time in Bed	366.5	mins.
Total Sleep Time	**331.0**	mins.
Total Wake Time	35.5	mins.
Sleep Efficiency	**90.3**	%

13

SLEEP STAGING				
Stage 1	38.0	mins.	11.5	%
Stage 2	180.5	mins.	54.5	%
Stage 3	0.5	mins.	0.1	%
Stage 4	63.5	mins.	19.1	%
REM	49.0	mins.	14.8	%

LATENCIES		
Latency to stage 1	**6.0**	mins.
Latency to stage 2	10.0	mins.
Latency to REM	**61.0**	mins.

WAKETIME		
Wake between sleep onset and sleep offset	28.0	mins.
Wake after sleep offset	1.5	mins.
Awakenings lasting 1-5 mins.	4	
Awakenings > 5 mins.	0	

SLEEP DISORDERED BREATHING
(by CPAP pressure level)

Pressure Level in cm. H2O	Total Time Pressure Administered (mins.)	Index of Obstructive Apneas (per hour of sleep)	Index of Hypopneas (per hour of sleep)	Index of Central Apneas (per hour of sleep)	Total Apnea/Hypopnea Index (per hour of sleep)
No Pressure	0.0	0.0	0.0	0.0	
5.0	82.8		6.4	0.0	6.4
7.5	283.8	0.0	2.3	0.0	2.3

14

BASELINE CARDIORESPIRATORY DATA

	Wake	REM	NREM
ECG	56-85	50-90	47-59
Respiratory Rate	12-14	14-24	10-14
SaO2*	99-100 %	97-100 %	96-98 %

FIGURE C7-8
CPAP report, page 1.

OTHER CARDIORESPIRATORY DATA

Body Position: The patient slept in the supine and, right and left lateral decubitus positions.

Undisturbed sleep: Approximately 2.3 hours.

Snoring: Did not occur with administration of NCPAP.

Arrhythmias: None

MOVEMENT PARAMETERS

15

	#	Index	
Total periodic leg movements in sleep (PLMS)	76	13.8	per hour of sleep
PLMS resulting in arousal	24	4.3	per hour of sleep
Duration of arousals	3-30	seconds	
Total nonperiodic leg movements in sleep (NPLMS)	0	0.0	per hour of sleep
NPLMS resulting in arousal			per hour of sleep
Duration of arousals		seconds	

ADDITIONAL FINDINGS

The patient reported on the AM questionnaire sleeping worse than usual.

MEDICATIONS

Type	Amount	When taken
None		

FIGURE C7-8
CPAP report, page 2.

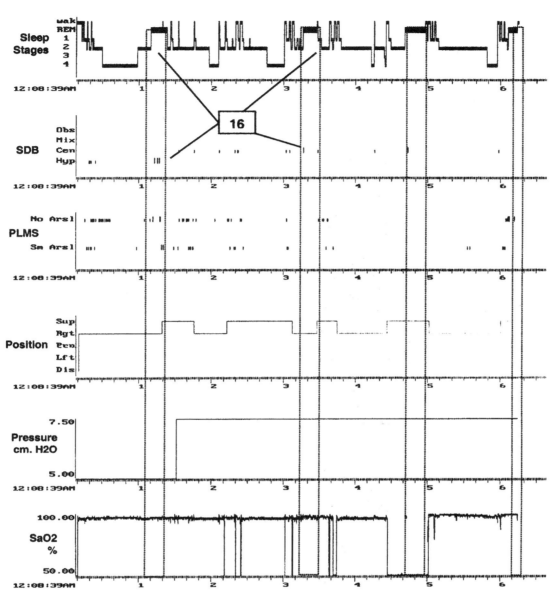

FIGURE C7-9
CPAP histogram.

3. Rebound deep sleep or REM sleep may represent sleep that is better in quality than will occur after several days or weeks of treatment. Therefore, the patient actually may be more alert on the day after the NCPAP treatment trial than at home.

4. Patients with moderate or severe obstructive sleep apnea and a secondary diagnosis of mild periodic leg movements in sleep (PLMS) find that, with successful treatment of sleep apnea, the PLMS may increase in both number and as a source of sleep fragmentation. PLMS may require pharmacotherapy before the patient's sleep quality approaches normal and daytime alertness improves significantly.

FOLLOW-UP PLAN

The diagnosis of narcolepsy has not been completely ruled out, even with the objectively successful administration of NCPAP. With an estimated incidence of sleep apnea of at least 4% in this patient's age group, sleep apnea certainly could occur concurrently with narcolepsy. Therefore, the patient will be followed using sleep logs for three to four weeks to determine if his subjective alertness improves. If there is significant improvement in alertness with NCPAP treatment, then further testing will be postponed or canceled. However, if subjective alertness is not improved over the baseline, then the patient will return to the sleep laboratory for a repeat nocturnal polysomnogram with administration of NCPAP at the optimal level throughout the recording. This will be followed by a standard MSLT.

Repeat Sleep Log (Figure C7-10)

17. This sleep log documents far fewer awakenings from sleep than noted on the previous sleep log.

18. There appears to be little or no difference in the number of short and long naps with CPAP treatment. Additionally, the patient continues to rate his fatigue as medium or high.

Polysomnogram with Administration of 7.5 cm H$_2$O

The results of this study were remarkably similar to those of the CPAP treatment trial and will not be repeated here.

Repeat Multiple Sleep Latency Test (Figure C7-11)

19. The mean sleep latency remains in the range of severe daytime sleepiness and shows only a minor difference from the previous MSLT. Three SOREMPs are present, demonstrating that successful CPAP treatment of this patient's sleep apnea had no obvious effects on the results.

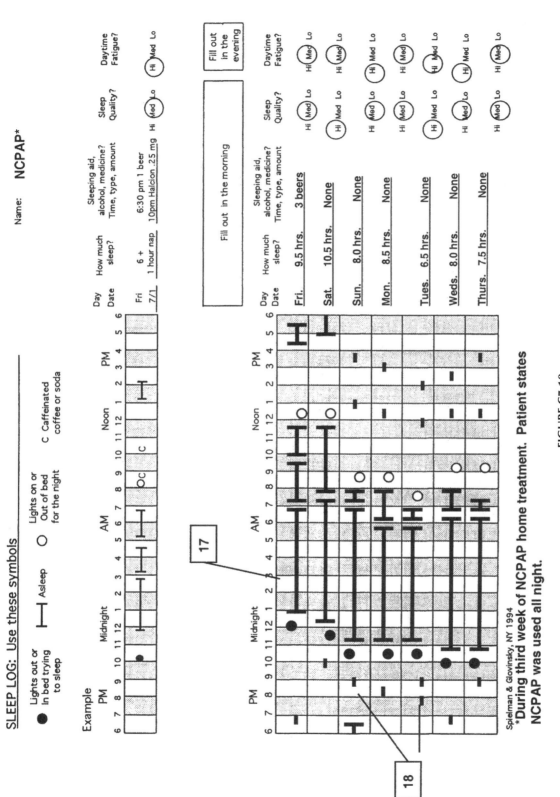

FIGURE C7-10

Sleep log before repeat MSLT.

MULTIPLE SLEEP LATENCY TEST (MSLT) REPORT

DESCRIPTION OF PROCEDURES: The MSLT consists of 5 twenty minute nap opportunities given at 2 hour intervals throughout the course of one day. Patients are instructed to fall asleep as quickly as possible. If sleep occurs the nap is terminated 15 minutes after sleep onset. Patients are not permitted to sleep between scheduled naps. All data are visually scored and analyzed according to standard criteria.

TEST RESULTS

LATENCIES (in minutes)						19
	10:00 AM	12:00 PM	2:00 PM	4:00 PM	6:00 PM	Mean
First signs of drowsiness	1.5	2.5	0.0	1.5	3.0	1.7
Latency to Stage 1	2.0	3.0	0.5	2.0	3.0	2.1
Latency to Stage 2	7.0	5.5	8.5	4.5	6.0	6.3
Latency to REM	3.0	5.0	-	2.5	-	

* A latency of 20 minutes indicates that no sleep occurred in the allotted time.

MEDICATIONS: None

20

ADDITIONAL DATA: The patient reported that he was as alert as usual during the day.

FIGURE C7-11
Repeat MSLT report.

FINAL SYNTHESIS

This case demonstrates that the process of determining final diagnoses can be long and complicated. At the end of this process, it was determined that narcolepsy was most likely the primary diagnosis and primary source of the patient's daytime sleepiness. Administration of CPAP resulted in little improvement in subjective or objective markers of daytime sleepiness. However, sleep apnea also was present and the likely source of other complaints that occur during the patient's sleep. Therefore, this patient is dually diagnosed and provided treatment for both disorders.

Case 8

PATIENT DEMOGRAPHICS

The patient is a 16-year-old male, high school sophomore.

PATIENT SLEEP HISTORY

For two years, the patient has been unable to fall asleep at a socially acceptable hour. He typically gets into bed by 11 PM but does not fall asleep until 4 AM. The patient reports only 4 hr of sleep on a typical school night. He will awaken twice for unknown reasons and is very groggy on awakening at 6:45 AM. On weekends, he gets into bed between 12 and 1 AM but does not fall asleep until 4 or 5 AM. He then sleeps for 8–10 hr, if permitted. During the period between lights out and sleep onset, the patient remains in bed in the dark. He reports ruminations and feelings of anxiety during that time. The patient denies snoring and restless legs.

The family history is positive for both an uncle and grandparent who occasionally have similar symptoms.

MEDICAL HISTORY AND EXAM

On examination the patient 5'8" and weighs 155 lbs. The physical examination was unremarkable. On in-terview, the patient appeared quite fatigued but motivated to solve his sleeping problems. He did not appear depressed, with no other signs of an affective disorder. However, he did relate that he was upset due to the separation of his parents in the past year.

PRELIMINARY DIAGNOSES

1. Delayed sleep phase syndrome—Common in adolescence; difficulty falling asleep, but sleep is normal once asleep; unable to awaken at socially acceptable times.
2. Psychophysiological insomnia—Significant rumination and feelings of anxiety.
3. Affective disorder—Separation of parents.

PLAN

Perform a diagnostic polysomnogram (DPSG) with special arrangements to allow patient to sleep to noon, if necessary.

COMMENTARY ON CLINICAL MATERIALS

All boxed numbers in the figures refer to the following comments.

Sleep Log

The patient did not fill out a sleep log as requested.

Bedtime Questionnaire (Figure C8-1)

1. The patient noted an estimated 2 hr sleep latency, shorter than reported during the initial office evaluation.

2. Thirty minutes before lights out (1:05 AM), the patient reported that he felt too alert to go to bed.

Diagnostic Polysomnogram (Figures C8-2 and C8-3)

3. At the patient's request lights out was postponed until after 1 AM. The patient awakened spontaneously at 7 AM and requested the study be ended.

4. During the slightly more than 5 hr of sleep recorded, a higher than expected quantity of REM sleep and deep sleep in the lower range of normal were recorded.

5. REM sleep latency was slightly shorter than expected.

6. A mild degree of sleep apnea was present, resulting in sleep fragmentation, primarily in the first third of the recording.

7. The sleep histogram is most remarkable for the reversed pattern of REM sleep period durations. Typically, the first REM sleep period is the shortest, with subsequent REM sleep periods increasing in duration. As noted here, the first REM sleep period is the longest in duration and subsequent REM sleep periods become progressively shorter. The usually reported sleep parameters are unable to document this phenomenon. Only examination of the sleep histogram can make this determination. This phenomenon of reversed pattern of REM sleep period durations has been reported during the sleep of depressed patients.[87]

Morning Questionnaire (Figure C8-4)

8. The patient noted on his AM questionnaire that he does not believe he slept at all. He informed the technologist that, since he had not slept, he might as well leave. Sleep state misperception is a common finding in insomnia.

Sample Interpretation

This recording is remarkable for the sleep-disordered breathing, REM sleep abnormalities, and sleep state misperception. A total of 49 apneas and hypopneas were noted during 316 min of recording, for an overall respiratory disturbance index (RDI) of 9.1/hr of sleep. Apneas and hypopneas generally were short in duration, averaging 16 sec, with occasional hypopneas during non-REM sleep, with durations 25 sec. Apneas and hypopneas generally were associated with minor O_2 desaturation, with 88% the lowest value noted. Low-volume rhythmic snoring was noted only with the patient in prone body position.

Sleep quantity was less than expected for a patient of this age but generally within normal limits except for REM sleep parameters. REM sleep percentage was higher than expected and REM sleep latency shorter than expected. These changes may represent REM sleep rebound. Additionally, the pattern of REM sleep periods across the night was quite unusual. Generally, the first REM sleep period is the shortest in duration with subsequent REM sleep periods increasing in duration. REM sleep during this study showed the opposite pattern, with the first REM sleep period having the longest duration and subsequent REM sleep periods becoming shorter and shorter. This reversed pattern of REM sleep period durations has been reported in patients with depression.

Although 5.3 hr of sleep were recorded, including good quantities of deep sleep and REM sleep, the patient reported that he did not sleep at all. The subjective underestimation of sleep most often is attributed to sleep state misperception. Sleep state misperception is an independent sleep disorder and a common feature of many types of insomnia.

In summary, these findings are consistent with the diagnosis of mild sleep apnea and suggestive of a diagnosis of depression and insomnia.

BEDTIME QUESTIONNAIRE

How sleepy do you feel right now? Place mark along line.

Very sleepy_____✕_____ Very Alert

Please describe how you feel now. Circle one of the numbers on the Stanford Sleepiness Scale below:

1. Alert. Wide Awake. Energetic.
2. Functioning at a high level, but not at peak. Able to concentrate.
3. Awake, but not fully alert.
4. A little foggy, let down.
5. Foggy. Beginning to lose interest in remaining awake. Slowed down.
6. Cannot stay awake. Sleep onset soon.

Please describe your sleep last night:

What time did you turn out the lights?	11:00 PM	
How long did it take to fall asleep?	120 minutes	1
How many hours/minutes did you sleep last night?	6 hrs.	
What time did you awaken this morning?	7 AM	
How many times did you awaken last night?	2	

Did you nap or fall asleep today?   Yes   (No)
If YES, please indicate at what times and for how long
_____

Was today a typical day?   (Yes)   No
If NO, please explain
_____

How well do you expect to sleep tonight?
Well
_____

Do you feel ready to go to sleep right now?   Yes   (No)   2
If NO, please explain
Too alert
_____

Did you drink any alcohol today?   Yes   (No)

If YES, please list what kind, how much and when taken
_____

Did you drink any caffeinated beverages (coffee, tea, colas, etc.) today? (YES) NO

FIGURE C8-1
Bedtime questionnaire, page 1.

If YES, please what kind, when taken and how much?
Iced tea with lunch
_____

Did you smoke any cigarettes, cigars, pipe, etc. today?   YES (NO)

If YES, please what kind, when taken and how much?

_____

Please list all medications you took today. Be sure to include prescriptions medications as well as those you take without a prescription

Name	How Much	Reason	When Taken
None			

Please list any other medication you will be taking before going to sleep

Name	How Much	Reason	When Taken
None			

Please list any other medication you have stopped taking in the last 30 days.

Name	How Much	Reason	When Taken
None			

Please describe anything else that occurred last night or today that might affect your sleep tonight. _____
_____

FIGURE C8-1
Bedtime questionnaire, page 2.

Lights out: 1:05 AM   Lights on: 7:04 AM

3

SLEEP PARAMETERS

GENERAL		
Total Time in Bed	358.0	mins.
Total Sleep Time	**316.0**	mins.
Total Wake Time	42.0	mins.
Sleep Efficiency	**88.3**	%

SLEEP STAGING				
Stage 1	21.5	mins.	6.8	%
Stage 2	118.5	mins.	37.5	%
Stage 3	7.0	mins.	2.2	%
Stage 4	51.5	mins.	16.3	%
REM	117.5	mins.	37.2	%

4

LATENCIES		
Latency to stage 1	8.5	mins.
Latency to stage 2	20.0	mins.
Latency to REM	70.0	mins.

WAKETIME		
Wake between sleep onset and sleep offset	14.0	mins.
Wake after sleep offset	19.5	mins.
Awakenings lasting 1-5 mins.	4	
Awakenings > 5 mins.	0	

5

SLEEP DISORDERED BREATHING

	Obstructive		Hypopnea		Central		Totals		
	REM	NREM	REM	NREM	REM	NREM	REM	NREM	All
# of apneas/hypopneas	0	0	12	20	6	10	18	30	49
Index (#/hr. of sleep)			2.2	3.8	1.1	1.9	9.1	9.0	9.1
Max. Duration (secs)			22.9	26.2	16.7	24.3			
Avg. Duration (secs.)			18.1	17.9	15.0	14.3			
Low SaO2 (%)			90.2	87.5	92.9	92.9			
Avg. SaO2 (%)			93.2	93.3	94.5	94.8			
Avg. Arousal (secs.)			7	21	4	11			

6

BASELINE CARDIORESPIRATORY DATA

	Wake		REM		NREM	
ECG	55-93		55-81		48-74	
Respiratory Rate	11-20		12-26		12-19	
SaO2*	97-100	%	92-95	%	93-97	%

*SaO2 measured by pulse oximeter.

FIGURE C8-2
Polysomnogram (DPSG) report, page 1.

OTHER CARDIORESPIRATORY DATA

Body Position: Sleep was recorded while in the left and right lateral decubitus, prone and supine positions.

Post Apnea/hypopnea arousals: Usually ranged 4-50 seconds.

Undisturbed sleep: Approximately 4 hours.

Snoring: Low volume rhythmic snoring occurred only while prone.

Arrhythmias: None

MOVEMENT PARAMETERS

	#	Index	
Total periodic leg movements in sleep (PLMS)	0	0	per hour of sleep
PLMS resulting in arousal			per hour of sleep
Duration of arousals	-	seconds	
Total nonperiodic leg movements in sleep (NPLMS)	0	0	per hour of sleep
NPLMS resulting in arousal			per hour of sleep
Duration of arousals	-	seconds	

ADDITIONAL FINDINGS

Patient reported at "lights on" that he felt like he hadn't slept at all.

MEDICATIONS

Type	Amount	When taken
None		

FIGURE C8-2
Polysomnogram (DPSG) report, page 2.

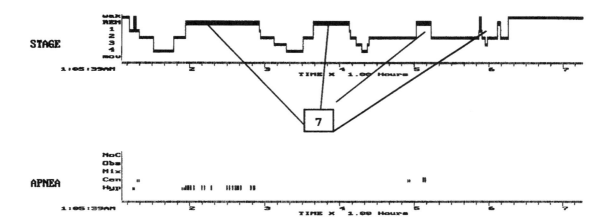

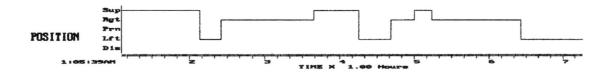

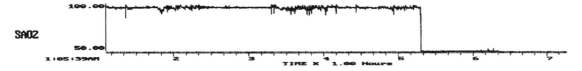

FIGURE C8-3
Polysomnogram (DPSG) histogram.

MORNING QUESTIONNAIRE

All things considered, your sleep last night was

(circle one answer)

1. Much better than usual
2. Better than usual
3. Same as usual
4. Worse than usual
5. Much worse than usual

Compared to the way you usually feel after awakening do you

1. Feel much more alert and awake than usual
2. Feel more alert and awake than usual
3. Feel same as usual
4. Feel less alert and awake than usual
5. Feel much less alert and wake than usual

How long did it take you to fall asleep last night? ___??___ mins.

Compared to the usual time it takes you to fall asleep, this was
1. Much shorter
2. Shorter
3. Same
4. Longer
5. Much longer

How many hours/minutes did you sleep last night? _0 hrs./mins*._____   8

Compared to the usual time you sleep at home, this was
1. Much longer
2. Longer
3. Same
4. Shorter
5. Much shorter

How many times did you awaken last night? _____??_ times

*Patient stated to technician that he did not recall sleeping at all.

FIGURE C8-4
Morning questionnaire.

FINAL SYNTHESIS

The initial clinical interview was strongly suggestive of a biological rhythm disorder—delayed sleep phase syndrome—common in patients of this age. The polysomnogram was ordered to document an expected very long sleep latency followed by otherwise normal sleep. Additionally, it was hoped that the polysomnogram would rule out other disorders.

The polysomnogram failed to provide objective confirmation for the preliminary diagnosis delayed sleep phase syndrome, characterized by difficulty falling asleep until 4 or 5 AM. The patient did not fall asleep until 1:15 AM, suggesting that only a 1–2 hr phase delay might be present. However, this shorter phase delay could be problematic during the school week, resulting in significant cumulative partial sleep deprivation.

The main findings of the recording were abnormalities in REM sleep and sleep state misperception. Taken together, these findings suggest a primary finding of insomnia and depression.

A last point is the importance of reviewing sleep data graphically, as presented in histograms. This presentation often allows a visual summation of the data, permitting rapid review. Additionally, it sometimes provides important information that cannot be found in the usual summary statistics.

References

1. Rechtshaffen A, Kales A. *A Manual of Standardized Terminology, Techniques, and Scoring System for Sleep Stages of Human Subjects.* Public Health Service Publication No. 204. Washington, DC: U.S. Government Printing Office, 1968.
2. Roehrs TA, Carskadon MA. Standardization of method: Essential to sleep science. *Sleep.* 1998;21(5):445.
3. Webb WB, Agnew HW. Sleep: Effects of a restricted regime. *Science.* 1965;150:1745–1747.
4. Bonnet MH. Performance and sleepiness as a function of frequency and placement of sleep disruption. *Psychophysiology.* 1986;23(3):263–271.
5. Stepanski E, Lamphere J, Roehrs T, Zorick F, Roth T. Experimental sleep fragmentation in normal subjects. *Int J Neuroscience.* 1994;33:207–214.
6. Bonnet MH. The effect of sleep fragmentation on sleep performance in younger and older subjects. *Neurobiol Aging.* 1989;10:21–25.
7. Roehrs T, Merlotti L, Petrucelli N, Stepanski E, Roth T. Experimental sleep fragmentation. *Sleep.* 1994;17:438–443.
8. Bonnet MH. Sleep restoration as a function of periodic awakening, movement, or electroencephalographic change. *Sleep.* 1987;10(4):364–373.
9. Martin SE, Engleman HM, Deary IJ, Douglas NJ. The effect of sleep fragmentation on daytime function. *Am J Respir Crit Care Med.* 1996;153:1328–1332.
10. Martin SE, Wraith PK, Deary IJ, Douglas NJ. The effect of nonvisible sleep fragmentation on daytime function. *Am J Respir Crit Care Med.* 1997;155:1596–1601.
11. Kader GA, Griffin PT. Reevaluation of the phenomena of the first night effect. *Sleep.* 1983;6(1):67–71.
12. Browman CP, Cartwright RD. The first-night effect on sleep and dreams. *Biological Psychiatry.* 1980;15(5):809–812.
13. Hauri PJ, Olmstead EM. Reverse first night effect in insomnia. *Sleep.* 1989;12(2):97–105.
14. Ware JC, Moorad PJ, Fanklin DB. Reduction of sleep apnea during stage 4 sleep. *Sleep Research.* 1981;10:241.
15. Carskadon MA, Wolfson AR, Acebo C, Tzischinsky O, Seifer R. Adolescent sleep patterns, circadian timing and sleepiness at a transition to early school days. *Sleep.* 1998;21(8):871–881.
16. Reynolds CF, Kupfer DJ, Buysse DJ, Coble PA, Yeager A. Subtyping DSM-III-R primary insomnia: A literature review by the DSM-IV Work Group on Sleep Disorders. *Am J Psychiat.* 1991;148(4):432–438.
17. McGregor P, Thorpy MJ, Schmidt-Nowara WW, Ledereich PS, Snyder M. T-sleep: An improved method for scoring breathing-disordered sleep. *Sleep.* 1992;15(4):359–363.
18. Halasz P, Pal I, Rajna P. K complex formation of the EEG in sleep. A survey and new examinations. *Acta Physiologica Hungarica.* 1985;65(1):3–35.
19. Takigawa M, Uchida T, Matsumoto K. [Correlation between occurrences of spontaneous K complex and the two physiological rhythms of cardiac and respiratory cycles]. [Japanese] *No to Shinkei—Brain and Nerve.* 1980;32(2):127–133.
20. Jankel WR, Niedermeyer E. Sleep spindles. *J Clin Neurophysiol.* 1985;2(1):1–35.
21. Azumi K, Shirakawa S. Characteristics of spindle activity and their use in evaluation of hypnotics. *Sleep.* 1982;5:95–105.
22. Johnson LC, Spinweber CL, Seidel WF, Dement WC. Sleep spindle and depth changes during chronic use of a short acting and long acting benzodiazepine hypnotic. *Electroencephalogr Clin Neurophysiol.* 1983;55:662–667.
23. Hirshkowitz M, Thornby JI, Karacan I. Sleep spindles pharmacological effects in humans. *Sleep.* 1982;5(1):85–94.
24. Feinberg I. Functional implications of changes in sleep physiology with age. In: Terry RD, Gershon S (eds.). *Neurobiology of Aging.* New York: Raven Press, 1976:23–41.
25. Bonnett MH, Arand DL. The consequences of a week of insomnia. *Sleep.* 1996;19(6):453–461.
26. Boselli M, Parrino L, Smerieri A, Terzano MG. Effect of age of EEG arousals in normal sleep. *Sleep.* 1998;21(4):351–357.
27. Marthur R, Douglas NJ. Frequency of EEG arousals from nocturnal sleep in normal subjects. *Sleep.* 1995;18(5):330–333.

28. Hauri P, Hawkins DR. Alpha-delta sleep. *Electroencephalogr Clin Neurophysiol.* 1973;34(3):233–237.

29. American Academy of Sleep Medicine Task Force, Flemons WW, Buysse D, cochairmen. Sleep related breathing in adults: Recommendations for syndrome definition and measurement techniques in clinical research. *Sleep.* 1999;22(5):667–689.

30. Littner MR, Shepard JW. Recommendations for research into measurement and classification of sleep disordered breathing: Gazing into a crystal ball. *Sleep.* 1999;22(5):665–666.

31. Young TM, Palta J, Dempsey J, Skatrud S, Weber T, Bade S. The occurrence of sleep-disordered breathing among middle-aged adults. *N Engl J Med.* 1993;328:1230–1235.

32. Young T, Blustein J, Finn L, Palta M. Sleep-disordered breathing and motor vehicle accidents in a population-based sample of employed adults. *Sleep.* 1997;20:608–613.

33. Young T, Peppard P, Palta M, Hla KM, Finn L, Morgan B, Skatrud J. Population-based study of sleep-disordered breathing as a risk factor for hypertension. *Arch Intern Med.* 1997;157:1746–1752.

34. Engleman HM, Kingshott RN, Wraith PK, Mackay TW, Deeary IJ, Douglas NJ. Randomized placebo controlled crossover trial of continuous positive airway pressure for mild sleep apnea/hypopnea syndrome. *Am J Respir Crit Care Med.* 1999;159:461–467.

35. Gall R, Isaac L, Krvger M. Quality-of-life in mild obstructive sleep apnea. *Sleep.* 1993;6:S59–S61.

36. Bedard MA, Montplaisir J, Malo J, Richler F, Rouleau I. Persistent neuropsychological deficits and vigilance impairment in sleep apnea syndrome after treatment with continuous positive airways pressure (CPAP). *J Clin Exp Neuropsychol.* 1993;15:330–341.

37. Kim HC, Young T, Matthews CG, Weber SM, Woodard AR, Palla M. Sleep-disordered breathing and neuropsychological deficits: A population-based study. *Am J Respir Crit Care Med.* 1997;156:1813–1819.

38. Redline S, Strauss SE, Adams N, Winters M, Roebuck T, Spry K, Rosenburg C, Adams K. Neuropsychological function in mild sleep-disordered breathing. *Sleep.* 1997;20:160–167.

39. Bedard MA, Montplaisir J, Richer F, Rouleau I, Malo J. Obstructive sleep apnea syndrome: Pathogenesis of neuropsychological deficits. *J Clin Exp Neuropsychol.* 1991;13:950–964.

40. Engleman HM, Martin SE, Deary IJ, Douglas NJ. The effect of continuous positive airway pressure therapy on daytime function in the sleep apnoea/hypopnoea syndrome. *Lancet.* 1994;343:572–575.

41. Fornas C, Ballester E, Arteta E, Ricou C, Diaz A, Fernandez A, Alonso J, Montserrat JM. Measurement of general health status in obstructive sleep apnea hypopnea patients. *Sleep.* 1995;18:876–879.

42. Gonzalez-Rothi RJ, Foresman GE, Block AJ. Do patients with sleep apnea die in their sleep? *Chest.* 1988;94(3):531–538.

43. Naegele B, Thouvard V, Pepin JL, Levy P, Bonnet C, Perret JE, Pellat J, Feuerstein C. Deficits of cognitive executive functions in patients with sleep apnea syndrome. *Sleep.* 1995;18:43–52.

44. Valencia-Flores M, Bliwise DL, Guilleminault C, Cilveti R, Clerk A. Cognitive function in patients with sleep apnea after acute nocturnal nasal continuous positive airway pressure (CPAP) treatment: Sleepiness and hypoxemia effects. *J Clin Exp Neuropsychol.* 1996;18:197–210.

45. Findley LJ, Unverzagt ME, Suratt PM. Automobile accidents involving patients with obstructive sleep apnea. *Am Rev Respir Dis.* 1988;138:337–340.

46. Placidi F, Diomedi M, Cupini LM, Bernardi G, Silvestrini M. Impairment of daytime cerebrovascular reactivity in patients with obstructive sleep apnoea syndrome. *J Sleep Res.* 1998;7(4):288–292.

47. Findley LJ, Fabrizio MJ, Knight H, Norcross BB, Laforte AJ, Suratt PM. Driving simulator performance in patients with sleep apnea. *Am Rev Respir Rev.* 1989;140:529–530.

48. Findley LJ, Barth JT, Powers DC, Wilhoit SC, Boyd DG, Suratt PM. Cognitive impairment in patients with obstructive sleep apnea and associated hypoxemia. *Chest.* 1986;90:686–690.

49. Stoneham MD. Uses and limitations of pulse oximetry. *Brit J Hosp Med.* 1995;54(1):35–41.

50. Webb RK, Ralston AC, Runciman WB. Potential errors in pulse oximetry. II: Effects of changes in saturation and signal quality. *Anaesthesia.* 1991;46:207–212.

51. Severinghaus JW, Kelleher JF. Recent developments in pulse oximetry. *Anesthesiology.* 1992;76:1018–1038.

52. Diagnostic Classification Steering Committee, Thorpy MJ, chairman. *International Classification of Sleep Disorders. Diagnostic and Coding Manual.* Rochester, MN: American Sleep Disorders Association, 1990.

53. Bethge K. Classification of arrhythmias. *J Cardiovascular Pharmacology.* 1991;17(suppl. 6):S13–S19.

54. Gregoratos G, Cheitlin MD, Conill A, Epstein AE, Fellows C, Ferguson TB, Freedman RA, Hlatky MA, Naccarelli GV, Saksena S, Schlant RC, Silka MJ. ACC/AHA guidelines for implantation of cardiac pacemakers and antiarrhythmia devices: A report of the American College of Cardiology/American Heart Association Task Force on Practice Guidelines (Committee on Pacemaker Implantation). *J Am Coll Cardiol.* 1998;31(5):1175–1209.

55. Mangrum JM, DiMarco JP. The evaluation and management of bradycardia. *N Engl J Med.* 2000;342(10):703–709.

56. Lown B, Wolf M. Approaches to sudden death from coronary heart disease. *Circulation.* 1971;44:130–142.

57. Metersky ML, Castriotta RJ. The effect of polysomnography on sleep position: Possible implications on the diagnosis of positional obstructive sleep apnea. *Respiration.* 1996;63(5):283–287.

58. Young T, Peppard P, Palta M, Hla KM, Finn L, Morgan B, Skatrud J. Population-based study of sleep-disordered breathing as a risk factor for hypertension. *Arch Intern Med.* 1997;157:1746–1752.

59. Indications for Polysomnography Task Force, Chesson A, chairman. Practice parameters for the indications for polysomnography and related procedures. *Sleep.* 1997;20(6):406–422.

60. Coleman R. Periodic movements in sleep (nocturnal myoclonus) and restless legs syndrome. In: Guilleminault C (ed). *Sleep and waking disorder: Indications and techniques.* Menlo Park, CA: Addison-Wesley, 1982:265–295.

61. Carskadon MA, Dement WC. Sleep loss in elderly volunteers. *Sleep.* 1985;8(3):207–221.

62. Browman CP, Gujavarty KS, Yolles SF, Mitler MM. Forty-eight-hour polysomnographic evaluation of narcolepsy. *Sleep.* 1986;9(1, Pt 2):183–188.

63. Roth T, Hartse KM, Zorick F, Conway W. Multiple naps and the evaluation of daytime sleepiness in patients with upper airway sleep apnea. *Sleep.* 1980;3:425–439.

64. Scrima L, Hartman PG, Johnson FH, Thomas EE, Hiller FC. The effects of gamma-hydroxybutyrate on the sleep of narcolepsy patients: A double-blind study. *Sleep.* 1990; 13(6):479–490.

65. Richardson G, Carskadon MA, Flagg W, van den Hoed J, Dement W, Mitler M. Excessive daytime sleepiness in man: Multiple sleep latency measurements in narcoleptic and control subjects. *Electroencephalogr Clin Neurophysiol.* 1978;45:621–627.

66. Zorick F, Roehrs T, Koshorek G, Sicklesteel J, Hartse K, Wittig R, Roth T. Patterns of sleepiness in various disorders of excessive daytime somnolence. *Sleep.* 1982;5:S165–S174.

67. Van de Hoed J, Kraemer H, Guilleminault C, Zarcone VP, Miles LE, Dement WC, Mitler MM. Disorders of excessive daytime sleepiness: Polygraphic and clinical data for 100 patients. *Sleep.* 1981;4:23–37.

68. Baker TL, Guilleminault C, Nino-Murcia G, Dement WC. Comparative polysomnographic study of narcolepsy and idiopathic central nervous system hypersomnia. *Sleep.* 1986;9(1, Pt 2):232–242.

69. Godbout R, Montplaisir J. All-day performance variations in normal and narcoleptic subjects. *Sleep.* 1986;9(1, Pt 2):200–204.

70. Roehrs T, Zorick F, Sickesteel J, Wittig R, Roth T. Excessive daytime sleepiness associated with insufficient sleep. *Sleep.* 1983;6(4):319–325.

71. Guilleminault C, Faull KF. Sleepiness in nonnarcoleptic, non-sleep apneic EDS patients: The idiopathic CNS hypersomnolence. *Sleep.* 1982;5:S175–S181.

72. Tafti M, Villemin E, Carlander B, Besset A, Billiard M. Sleep onset REM episodes in narcolepsy: REM sleep pressure or non-REM-REM sleep dysregulation. *J Sleep Res.* 1991;1(4):245–250.

73. Reynolds CF, Cobel PA, Kupfer DJ, Holzer BC. Application of multiple sleep latency test in disorders of exces-

sive sleepiness. *Electroencephalogr Clin Neurophysiol.* 1982; 53(4):443–452.

74. Carskadon MA, Seidel WF, Greenblatt DJ, Dement WC. Daytime carryover of triazolam and flurazepam in elderly insomniacs. *Sleep.* 1982;5(4):361–371.

75. Lumley M, Roehrs T, Asker D, Zorick F, Roth T. Ethanol and caffeine effects on daytime sleepiness/alertness. *Sleep.* 1987;10(4):306–312.

76. Pressman MR, Fry JM. Relationship of autonomic nervous system activity to daytime sleepiness and prior sleep. *Sleep.* 1989;12(3):239–245.

77. Bliwise D, Seidel W, Karacan I, Mitler M, Roth T, Zorick F, Dement W. Daytime sleepiness as a criterion in hypnotic medication trials: Comparison of triazolam and flurazepam. *Sleep.* 1983;6(2):156–163.

78. Roehrs T, Timms V, Zwyghuizen-Doorenbos A, Roth T. Sleep extension in sleep and alert normals. *Sleep.* 1989; 12(5):449–457.

79. Seidel WF, Ball S, Cohen S, Patterson N, Yost D, Dement WC. Daytime alertness in relation to mood, performance and nocturnal sleep in chronic insomniacs and noncomplaining sleepers. *Sleep.* 1984;7(3):230–238.

80. Clodore M, Benoit O, Foret J, Bouard G, The Multiple Sleep Latency Test: Individual variability and time of day effect in normal young adults. *Sleep.* 1990;13(5):385–394.

81. Levine B, Roehrs T, Stepanski E, Zorick F, Roth T. Fragmenting sleep diminishes its recuperative value. *Sleep.* 1987;10(6):590–599.

82. Stepanski E, Zorick F, Roehrs T, Young D, Roth T. Daytime alertness in patients with chronic insomnia compared with asymptomatic control subjects. *Sleep.* 1988; 11(1):54–60.

83. Seidel WF, Dement WC. Sleepiness in insomnia: evaluation and treatment. *Sleep.* 1982;5:S182–S190.

84. Palm L, Persson E, Elmqvist D, Blennow G. Sleep and wakefulness in normal preadolescent children. *Sleep.* 1989;12(4):299–308.

85. Aldrich MS, Chervin RD, Malow B. Value of the multiple sleep latency test for the diagnosis of narcolepsy. *Sleep.* 1997;20(8):620–629.

86. Bishop C, Rosenthal L, Helmus T, Roehrs T, Roth T. The frequency of multiple sleep onset REM periods among subjects with no excessive daytime sleepines. *Sleep.* 1996; 19(9):727–730.

87. Vogel GW, Vogel F, McAbee RS, Thurmond AJ. Improvement of depression by REM sleep deprivation. *Arch Gen Psychiatry.* 1980;37:247–253.

Index

Page references followed by "t" denote tables; "f" denote figures.

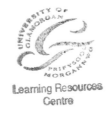